ESSENTIAL STATISTICS
FOR MEDICAL
EXAMINATIONS

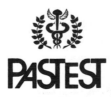

PASTEST

ESSENTIAL STATISTICS FOR MEDICAL EXAMINATIONS

Chris Marguerie MRCP
Consultant Physician, Consultant
Rheumatologist, Warwick Hospital, Warwick.

E Brian Faragher PhD FSS
Medical Statistics Research Support Unit,
University of Manchester, Manchester.

© 1998 PASTEST
Egerton Court
Parkgate Estate
Knutsford
Cheshire WA16 8DX

First published 1998

ISBN 0 906896 82 7

A catalogue record for this book is available from the British Library.

The information contained within this book was obtained by the authors from reliable sources. However, while every effort has been made to ensure its accuracy, no responsibility for loss, damage or injury occasioned to any person acting or refraining from action as a result of information contained herein can be accepted by the publishers or authors.

PasTest Revision Books and Intensive Courses

PasTest has been established in the field of postgraduate medical education since 1972, providing revision books and intensive study courses for doctors preparing for their professional examinations.

Books and courses are available for the following specialties: **MRCP Part 1 and Part 2 (General Medicine and Paediatrics), MRCOG, DRCOG, MRCGP, DCH, FRCA, MRCS, PLAB.**

For further details contact:

PasTest, Freepost, Knutsford, Cheshire WA16 7BR
Tel: 01565 755226   Fax: 01565 650264

Typeset by Breeze Limited, Manchester.
Printed by MPG Books Limited, Bodmin.

CONTENTS

Contents

RECOMMENDED READING LIST

An Introduction to Medical Statistics: Bland M, 2nd edition, Oxford University Press, 1995.

Clinical Trials: *A Practical Approach*: Pocock S J, Wiley, 1983.

Epidemiological Studies: *A Practical Guide*: Silman A J, Cambridge University Press, 1996.

Medical Statistics: *A Common Sense Approach*: Campbell M J and Machin D, 2nd edition, Wiley, 1993.

Practical Statistics for Medical Research: Altman D G, Chapman and Hall, 1990.

Statistics at Square One: Swinscow T D V and Campbell M J, 9th edition, BMJ Publishing Group, 1996.

Statistics with Confidence: Gardner M J and Altman D G, BMJ Publishing Group, 1989.

PREFACE

The purpose of this book is to help candidates to prepare for medical examinations. The material presented has been selected to cover those aspects of statistical methodology commonly tested by medical examiners.

A knowledge of statistics is <u>not</u> assumed. The essential concepts underlying statistical methods are summarised, their limitations are outlined and the situations in which they may be applied are described. Formulae for calculating statistics are included only if these aid in understanding the basic concepts involved. The mathematical content of this book is minimal.

This is not a substitute for a textbook on medical statistics. There are many excellent texts on this subject already available, a short list of those particularly recommended is included in the reading list on page viii. At least one of these should be used by anyone planning to apply statistical methods to real data.

A series of multiple choice questions similar to those set by the Royal College Examination Boards in their examinations is provided. A section on how to tackle a critical reading paper is also included.

The authors would like to thank Mr R. K. Harrison for providing the cartoons.

We are always grateful for notification of any mistakes or discrepancies that appear in our books. If you do find an item which you suspect may be incorrect please notify the Publisher in writing so that we can ensure that any mistake is rectified when the book is reprinted.

1: BASIC CONCEPTS AND DEFINITIONS

1.1 Why are statistics necessary?

> MEASUREMENTS OBTAINED FROM BIOLOGICAL SYSTEMS ARE
> INHERENTLY VARIABLE

In the following experiments, blood pressure readings were taken under identical conditions:

Experiment 1: all readings were taken from the <u>same</u> healthy individual on different days.

Experiment 2: readings were taken from <u>different</u> healthy individuals on the same day.

Experiment 3: readings were taken from several <u>different</u> individuals; some were taking a drug which reduces blood pressure, the rest were not.

A range of values were obtained in all three experiments. We would expect the range of values to be smallest in Experiment 1 and greatest in Experiment 3.

> Observations on the same individual under identical conditions are called replicates. Differences between replicate observations are due to random variation.
> Differences between observations which are due to the action of some known factors (such as the effect of a drug) are called systematic variation.

In the above three experiments, the range of values obtained will be due to:

Experiment 1: random variation only.

Experiment 2: a combination of random variation and a single source of systematic variation (inherent differences in blood pressure levels between individuals).

Experiment 3: a combination of random variation and two sources of systematic variation (inherent individual differences and the effect of the drug).

> STATISTICS IS THE SCIENCE OF ESTIMATING THE SOURCES OF
> VARIATION PRESENT IN AN EXPERIMENT

The estimated influence of a specific factor (such as the effect of a drug on blood pressure) can be compared with the estimated amount of random variation present. Doing so allows an informed decision to be made about whether the effect observed is likely to be:
- the result of systematic variation (i.e. a 'real' effect), or
- merely due to chance (random variation).

STATISTICAL CONSIDERATIONS ARE VITALLY IMPORTANT WHEN AN EXPERIMENT IS BEING PLANNED

A badly designed clinical trial may produce:
- **inadequate estimates** of a source of systematic variation
  (the study may not be powerful enough to detect the 'real' effect of a therapy)
- **confounding**
  (the effect of a factor of specific interest may be indistinguishable from that of some other, unmeasured factor; e.g. the 'real' effect of an anti-hypertensive drug would not be estimable if, on entering the study, patients were also advised to make changes in their life-style known to reduce blood pressure)
- **bias**
  (a study sample of unrepresentative individuals – see also section 1.2).

A poor or invalid statistical analysis can be repeated using correct methods. However, **no amount of data manipulation can compensate for flaws in the study design.**

Potential sources of systematic variation must be identified and incorporated into the study design. Otherwise, the results obtained may be distorted. If this happens, invalid or misleading conclusions may be drawn.

Example
In Experiment 3, the sphygmomanometer used for the patients receiving the drug gave results consistently 5 mmHg lower than the one used for the control group. Invalid conclusions would be drawn if this source of systematic variation was not detected. The study must be designed in such a way that the source of systematic variation is either:
- eradicated (the same sphygmomanometer is used for both groups), or
- balanced out (equal numbers of subjects in both groups are measured using each machine).

1.2 Populations and samples

Clinical studies usually involve samples of humans (patients, volunteers), a fact reflected throughout this book in the choice of illustrative examples. The material presented, however, applies equally to other types of experiment, such as animal and laboratory based studies. Ideally, a study should be conducted on all individuals with the characteristic of interest (*experimental units*) in a defined (*finite*) population. This is rarely possible. Instead, a random sample of individuals is usually selected for study. It is vital that the sample selected is *representative*. Otherwise, the results obtained cannot be extrapolated to the target population.

> The **target population** is the group of all individuals to whom the conclusions of the study will be applied (e.g. all patients with mild hypertension).
> The **study population** is the group of all individuals actually available for study – usually a limited, accessible subgroup of the target population (e.g. all patients with mild hypertension attending the clinics conducting the study).

A representative sample:
- truly reflects the variations (*random and systematic*) within the target population
- can usually be obtained by choosing a sufficiently large *random sample*
- is selected in such a way that every individual (*experimental unit*) in the study population has an equal chance of being chosen.

The characteristics of a properly selected random sample will be similar to, but not necessarily identical to, those of the target population. Several random samples drawn from the same study population will also have similar, but not identical, characteristics.

> DIFFERENCES BETWEEN RANDOM SAMPLES DRAWN FROM THE SAME POPULATION ARE DUE TO SAMPLING VARIATION

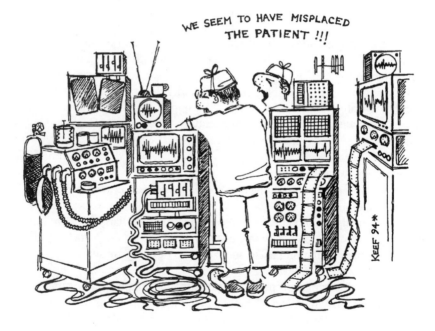

1.3 Types of statistical methods

Statistical analyses take many different forms, depending on the objectives of the study.

Descriptive statistics are used to summarise the observations from an experiment. They are usually computed in either of two situations:
- for a particular measure at a specific time (e.g. blood pressure before starting treatment)
- for a difference (e.g. change in blood pressure during a period of treatment).

Typically, a *central* (average) value is stated together with a measure of the *dispersion* (spread) of the observations around the central value.

Significance tests are used to assess the extent to which the observations from an experiment support (or refute) two stated propositions.

These take the form of a:
- **Null hypothesis**: usually a statement of 'no effect' (e.g. the changes in blood pressure observed during the treatment period were merely due to random variation)
- **Alternative hypothesis**: usually a statement of 'real effect' (e.g. the changes in blood pressure observed were systematic, in which case it may be reasonable to infer that they were a consequence of the drug taken).

A significance test is used to decide which hypothesis is accepted and which is rejected.

Measures of association are used to estimate the degree and nature of any (mathematical) relationship existing between two variables (measures).

1.4 Types of data

The exact nature of a statistical analysis depends on the nature of the observations obtained. The measures (*variables*) recorded in an experiment can be divided into two types, requiring the use of different statistical methods.

Qualitative variables are measures which are categorical. They classify individuals into distinct groups which often have no obvious numerical

relationship (e.g. blood group, sex). Numbers are attached to each of the categories to provide labels:
- *Nominal* variables have numbers allocated to the categories arbitrarily
  e.g. gender: 0 = male, 1 = female
- *Ordinal* variables use numbers which indicate an inherent ranking across the categories
  e.g. pain severity: 0 = nil, 1 = mild, 2 = moderate, 3 = severe.

Quantitative variables are measurements which are numerical, with the properties that:
- the values obtained are based on an *interval/continuous* scale
- the distance between adjacent values is constant and has a physical interpretation
- *discrete* variables are integers (whole numbers) and are usually counts
  e.g. number of asthmatic attacks suffered by a patient during a study
- *continuous* variables can (theoretically) take any value within a specific range, e.g. height, weight, drug concentration.

1.5 Accuracy and precision

All types of measurement share several important properties.

> **Accuracy** indicates how close a measurement is to the true value.
> **Precision** indicates how close replicate values are to each other; an instrument has 'high precision' if it produces values under constant conditions which vary minimally.

Example
Four different assays were used to measure haemoglobin (g/dl) in a blood sample taken from a patient. The correct haemoglobin value was known to be 11.0 g/dl.

Assay	Replicate measurements	Average	Accuracy	Precision
A	10.9 10.9 11.0 11.1 11.1	11.0	High	High
B	10.4 10.7 10.8 11.3 11.8	11.0	High	Low
C	10.3 10.3 10.4 10.5 10.5	10.4	Low	High
D	10.9 11.2 11.3 11.8 12.3	11.5	Low	Low

A method is *valid* if it measures what it purports to be measuring, e.g. the validity of a non-invasive diagnostic test could be tested by comparing the test result with that from a (often invasive) 'gold standard' such as a blood sample, biopsy or post-mortem. Validity is frequently impossible to determine directly and has to be assessed indirectly.

2.1 Qualitative variables

> QUALITATIVE DATA ARE OFTEN BEST DISPLAYED GRAPHICALLY
> USING EITHER A PIE DIAGRAM OR A BAR CHART

Example (Figs. 1a and 1b)
A sample of 1000 patients with arthritis were entered into a study; 500 had osteoarthritis, 350 had rheumatoid arthritis and 150 had psoriatic arthritis. The results of this study are shown as a pie diagram (Fig. 1a) and a bar chart (Fig. 1b).

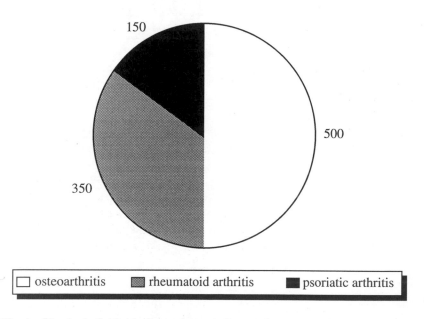

Fig. 1a: Pie chart of arthritis diagnosis group frequencies

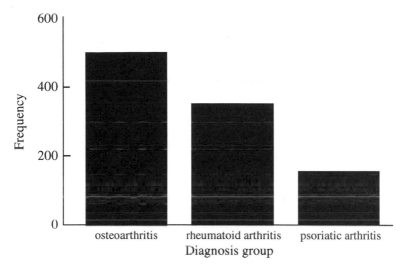

Fig. 1b: Bar chart of arthritis diagnosis group frequencies

2.2 Quantitative data

A variety of graphical methods exist for displaying quantitative data.

Dot diagrams show the distribution of the observations obtained from different subject groups by displaying each individual data point.

Example
A new biochemical test has been devised for helping in the diagnosis of a disease. Test results were obtained for a group of 44 patients known not to have the disease and 36 patients in whom the diagnosis was certain. The results of this study are shown in the form of a dot diagram in Fig. 2.

9

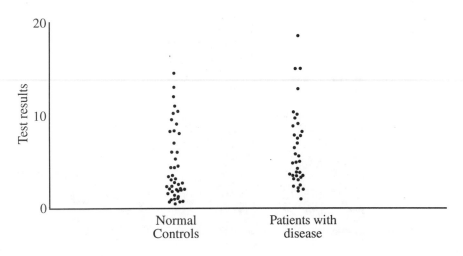

Fig. 2: Dot diagram

Placing the dot diagrams adjacently on the same scale shows that:
* the test result tends to be fractionally higher for patients with the disease
* the overlap between the groups is too great for the method to provide on its own a clinically useful diagnostic test.

Histograms show a series of bars, each bar corresponding to a particular range of test results. The *area* of the bar represents the number (or percentage) of patients within that range. Usually, all bars are given the same width, so that the *length* of the bar represents the number (or percentage) of patients with a result within a particular range.

Example (Fig. 3)
Measurements of inflamed joints were taken from 150 patients with psoriatic arthritis. The height of each histogram bar represents the number of patients with a particular number of affected joints. Four patients had just one swollen joint, eight had two swollen joints, and so on.

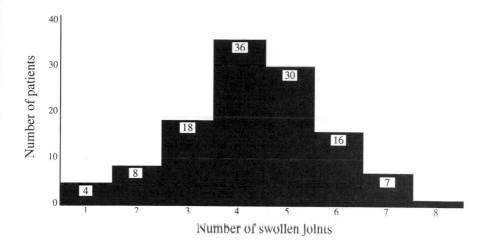

Fig. 3: Histogram - number of psoriatic arthritis patients with one or more swollen joints

Histograms appear deceptively simple. The rules concerning their construction are more complex than suggested in this example. A more detailed text should be consulted before attempting to create one.

Frequency distributions also show the number of times (frequency with which) a particular test result occurs. In this type of graph only the tops of the histogram bars are shown. These are joined to produce a (smooth) curve. **If drawn using percentages rather than frequencies on the vertical axis, the graph produced is called a *relative frequency distribution*.**

Example (Fig. 4)
The numbers of inflamed joints in the group of 150 patients with psoriatic arthritis (Fig. 3) are shown as a frequency distribution.

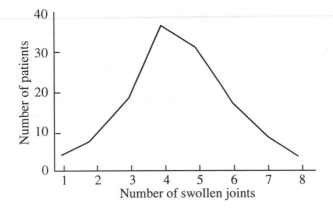

Fig. 4: Frequency distribution - number of psoriatic arthritis patients with one or more swollen joints

The information in a frequency distribution curve can be summarised by indicating:
- the middle of the data (*measure of central tendency/average*)
- the extent to which the individual observations are spread (distributed) around the mid-value (*measure of dispersion/variation*).

3.1 Definitions

Qualitative measures of the efficacy of a treatment take forms such as:
- patient response (cured/not cured)
- survival (alive/dead)
- the result of a diagnostic test (positive/negative)
- the severity of any side-effects experienced (nil/mild/moderate/severe).

The frequency with which each category occurs in an appropriately designed clinical trial provides an estimate of the efficacy of the treatment.

> The **probability** that an event will occur is the proportion of times the event happens in a (long) series of trials/experiments

There are two types of probability:
- **a *priori*** : the probability is determined theoretically.
  20 patients are to be selected for a study from 80 patients attending an out-patient clinic by drawing names at random.
  The probability of an individual patient being selected is 20/80 = 0.25 (or 25%).
- **a *posteriori*** : the probability is determined empirically.
  In a clinical trial, 30 of the 50 patients allocated to a new treatment were classified as having recovered.
  The probability of recovery for this treatment is estimated as 30/50 = 0.60 (or 60%).

3.2 Properties of probability

An analgesic was given pre-operatively to 300 patients having wisdom teeth extractions under a general anaesthetic. They were asked to rate the severity of their post-operative pain using the scale:

nil/mild/moderate/severe

The observed frequencies and (*a posteriori*) probabilities for the four categories were:

Category	nil	mild	moderate	severe
Frequency	15	90	120	75
Probability	15/300 = 0.05	90/300 = 0.30	120/300 = 0.40	75/300 = 0.25

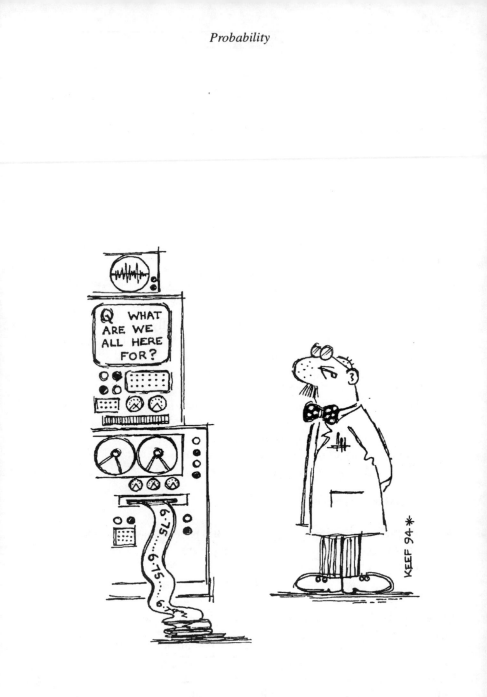

The sum of the probabilities of all possible categories is always equal to 1:

prob(nil) + prob(mild) + prob(moderate) + prob(severe)
= 0.05 + 0.30 + 0.40 + 0.25 = 1

Probability takes values between 0 and 1 inclusive:

* the probability is 0 if the category is reported by no patients (i.e. <u>never</u> happens)
* the probability is 1 if the category is reported by every patient (i.e. <u>always</u> happens)
* the best estimate of the probability of mild post-operative pain was 0.30 (30%) (on average, this will be recorded by 30 out of every 100 patients treated pre-operatively with the study analgesic).

As a patient could select only one point on the scale, the categories are **mutually exclusive**. The probability that a patient will record either of two mutually exclusive categories is the **sum** of the individual probabilities:

prob(moderate <u>or</u> severe) = prob(moderate) + prob(severe)
= 0.40 + 0.25 = 0.65 (65%)

As the category recorded by one patient could not be influenced by the category recorded by any other patient, the study events are **independent**.

The probability of two independent events occurring is the **product** of the two individual probabilities.

prob(patient A scores moderate <u>and</u> patient B scores severe) =
prob(A scores moderate) x prob(B scores severe) =
0.40 x 0.25 = 0.10 (10%)

3.3 Prevalence and incidence

The <u>total number</u> of individuals in a population with a particular characteristic (e.g. disease) at a given time is called the *point prevalence*.

point prevalence = number of existing cases in the population

The <u>proportion</u> of individuals with the characteristic at a given time is the *prevalence rate* (usually expressed as the number of cases per 100,000 individuals in the population).

> rate = (number of cases in population / total size of population) x 100,000

The total number of new individuals in a population presenting with a particular characteristic (e.g. new cases of a disease or condition) in a fixed period of time (usually one year) is called the *incidence*.

> incidence = number of new cases in the population per unit of time

The proportion of individuals in the population presenting with the characteristic in a fixed period of time is the *incidence rate* (again, usually expressed as the number of new cases per 100,000 individuals in the population).

> rate = (number of new cases / total size of population at risk) x 100,000

These two concepts are discussed again in greater detail in Chapter 8.

3.4 Sensitivity and specificity

> THE EXTENT TO WHICH A DIAGNOSTIC TEST CAN DISTINGUISH BETWEEN PATIENTS WITH AND WITHOUT A PARTICULAR DISEASE IS QUANTIFIED BY ITS **SENSITIVITY** AND **SPECIFICITY**

Sensitivity is the proportion of patients with the disease for whom the test is positive (the probability that the test will be positive when the disease is present).

Specificity is the proportion of patients without the disease for whom the test is negative (the probability that the test will be negative when the disease is absent).

Positive predictive value is the proportion of positive tests for which the disease is confirmed (the probability of a patient with a positive test result having the disease).

Negative predictive value is the proportion of negative tests for which the disease is found to be absent (the probability of a patient with a negative test result not having the disease).

POSITIVE AND NEGATIVE PREDICTIVE VALUES BOTH DIFFER
ACCORDING TO THE PREVALENCE OF THE DISEASE

SENSITIVITY AND SPECIFICITY ARE BOTH UNAFFECTED BY
DISEASE PREVALENCE

A diagnostic test is:
- 100% specific if there are no false positive results
- 100% sensitive if there are no false negative results.

There is always a trade off between sensitivity and specificity; as one increases, the other decreases (or, at best, remains unchanged).

Example
175 in-patients awaiting minor surgery were interviewed by a psychiatrist and then completed a simple questionnaire. Each patient was diagnosed as clinically 'anxious' or 'not anxious' on the basis of both the psychiatric interview ('true' diagnosis) and the questionnaire test score ('test' diagnosis).

		'True' diagnosis		Totals
		Anxious	Not anxious	
'Test' diagnosis	Anxious	55	7	62
	Not anxious	14	99	113
Totals		69	106	175

Sensitivity	= 55/69	= 0.797	(79.7%)
Specificity	= 99/106	= 0.934	(93.4%)
Positive predictive value	= 55/62	= 0.887	(88.7%)
Negative predictive value	= 99/113	= 0.876	(87.6%)

N.B. Clinical context usually determines whether the sensitivity or specificity of a test is most important. For example, when using a screening test for neonatal hypothyroidism or phenylketonuria, a number of false positives can be accepted but false negatives (missed diagnoses) would lead to the failure to treat the conditions early, with irreversible consequences.

4.1 Qualitative/categorical data

Frequency counts (the number of observations in each category) constitute a comprehensive summary of a qualitative variable.

<u>Example</u> Numbers of patients with arthritis falling into each of three diagnostic groups:

Diagnosis:	Osteoarthritis	Rheumatoid arthritis	Psoriatic arthritis
Number of patients:	500	350	150

Frequency counts do not always readily demonstrate the size of group differences.

<u>Example</u> Numbers of patients responding to two treatments in a comparative clinical trial:

Treatment group	Responders	Non-responders	Total sample
A	12	15	27
B	15	17	32

The response rates are clearly similar, but the size of the numerical difference between the treatments is not immediately obvious. To aid interpretation in such situations, frequency counts are often presented also as percentages (or *proportions*).

Treatment group	Number of responders	Number of non-responders	Total sample
A	12 (44%)	15 (56%)	27
B	15 (47%)	17 (53%)	32

Percentages/proportions should be used cautiously, as they can inadvertently mislead.

<u>Example</u> The response rate to a standard treatment is known to be 25%. A report of a recent clinical trial claims that the response rate for a new treatment was 80%. The statistical <u>and</u> clinical strength of this claim differs according to whether:
- 4 patients responded in a study of 5 patients, or

- 800 patients responded in a study of 1000 patients.

Percentages and proportions must always be reported with their raw frequency counts.

4.2 Quantitative data

Quantitative data (e.g. blood pressure, haemoglobin level, etc.) are best described by giving measures of both central tendency (**average**) and dispersion (**variation**).

4.2.1 Measures of central tendency

Three measures of central tendency are commonly used in medical statistics:

mean (arithmetic average): sum of the observations divided by the number of observations)
median: value which divides the observations into two equal halves when they are arranged in order of increasing value
mode: value which occurs most often

<u>Example</u>   Numbers of attacks reported by 15 migraine sufferers over a three month study period: 1 1 1 1 1 1 2 $2^{\dagger}$ 2 3 3 4 4 7 12

mean = $(1 + 1 + 1 + 1 + 1 + 1 + 2 + 2 + 2 + 3 + 3 + 4 + 4 + 7 + 12) / 15$
        = $45/15 = 3$
median = 2 (the observation identified by the symbol $\dagger$)
mode = 1

The **mode** is rarely used in practice:
- with small data sets, it can be difficult to estimate, as many different values may occur with equal frequency
- some data distributions naturally have several modal values
- if there are two such values the distribution is said to be *bimodal* (e.g. Fig. 5).

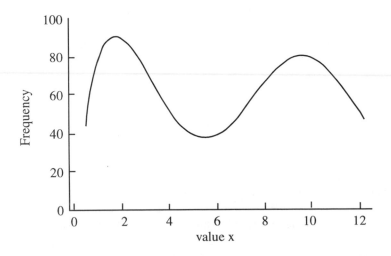

Fig. 5: Bimodal frequency distribution

4.2.2 Measures of dispersion (variation)

Variance
Intuitively, a good measure of dispersion would be the average amount each observation differs (deviates) from the mean value.

The <u>deviations</u> of the observations are defined as follows:
deviation of observation 1 = d_1 = mean value minus value of observation 1
deviation of observation 2 = d_2 = mean value minus value of observation 2
etc.

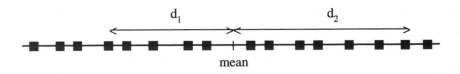

The <u>average deviation</u> is the arithmetic mean of these d values.
Unfortunately, this mean is always zero because the positive and negative values of d cancel each other out exactly!

This problem is resolved by summing the <u>squares</u> of the values of d. Squares cannot be negative. When summed, they must give a value greater than or equal to zero.

This statistic:
- is called the **sum of squares about the mean** (often shortened to **sum of squares**)
- measures only the size and not the direction of the deviations
- is determined by the amount of scatter in the data <u>and</u> the number of observations.

> The **variance** is defined as the average squared deviation. For mathematical reasons, this is obtained by dividing the sum of squares by the number of observations (n) minus 1 when estimated from a sample*.
> **Variance = (sum of squares about the mean)/(n – 1)**
> The units of the variance are the units of the variable squared.
> The quantity (n – 1) is called the **degrees of freedom** of the variance estimate.

Standard deviation

A measure of dispersion with the same units as both the observations and the sample mean is provided by the **standard deviation**, calculated by taking the square root of the variance:

> **Standard deviation = square root of variance**
> The standard deviation can be regarded as being approximately equal to the average distance each individual observation lies away from the sample mean.

Coefficient of variation

If several methods for measuring the same entity (e.g. laboratory assays) have different units, comparison of their precisions can be difficult. In this situation, the ratio of the standard deviation and mean is often used.

---

* n is used instead of (n - 1) only if the whole population has been studied.

This statistic:
- is usually expressed as a percentage
- has no units
- is called the **coefficient of variation**

(C.V.) = (standard deviation/mean) x 100.

Quantiles

Values which subdivide a continuous distribution into sections each containing specific proportions of the distribution are called **quantiles**. There are three important types.

- The quantile which divides a distribution into two equal parts is the **median**.
  The sections either side of the median both contain 50% (half) of the distribution.

- The three quantiles which divide a distribution into four equal parts are called **quartiles**.
  The first (lower) quartile is often referred to as Q25.
  The second (middle) quartile is the median.
  The third (upper) quartile is often referred to as Q75.
  The distance between the lower and upper quartiles is called the **interquartile range.**
  The four sections defined by the quartiles each contain 25% (a quarter) of the distribution.

- The quantiles which divide a distribution into 100 equal parts are called **percentiles.**
  The sections defined by the percentiles each contain 1% of the distribution.

Range

The simplest measure of dispersion for any variable is the range; i.e. the difference between the smallest and largest observation values.

5.1 Binomial distribution

There are many situations in which the outcome of an experiment has only two possibilities (e.g. cure/no cure, alive/dead, result positive/negative).

> QUALITATIVE MEASURES WHICH HAVE ONLY TWO POSSIBILITIES ARE CALLED **BINARY VARIABLES**
>
> THE RESULTS OF EXPERIMENTS INVOLVING BINARY VARIABLES CAN EASILY BE SUMMARISED AS PROPORTIONS OR PROBABILITIES

Example
The efficacy of a treatment for cancer of the stomach was determined by the proportion (p) of patients categorised as 'cured' in a study where a large number of patients with the condition were given the treatment. The value p can be interpreted as the (estimated) probability that a patient with stomach cancer will respond to the treatment.

Several new random samples of patients with this condition are now selected.
Each new patient will:
*   constitute an *independent* event
*   have the same theoretical probability of being cured.

Because of the effects of random variation, the actual proportion categorised as 'cured' will vary from sample to sample. The nature of this variation can be determined theoretically.

Using the rules outlined in section 3.2, the probabilities that given numbers of patients in a sample will be cured can be computed. These probabilities form a *probability distribution*.

> THE PROBABILITY DISTRIBUTION FOR A BINARY VARIABLE IS CALLED A **BINOMIAL DISTRIBUTION**

Fig. 6 shows three binomial distributions for a group of 20 patients. The first graph assumes a cure rate of $p = 0.25$; the second graph assumes a cure rate of 0.50; the third graph assumes a cure rate of $p = 0.75$.

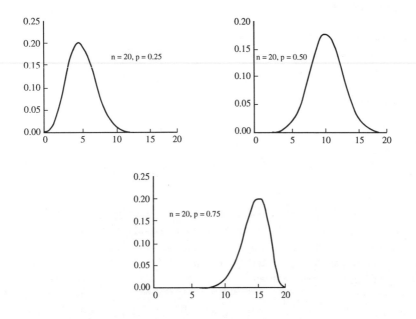

Fig. 6: Three examples of the binomial distribution

The exact shape of this distribution depends on the value of *the parameter* p:
• as p gets smaller, the binomial distribution becomes increasingly positively skewed
• as p gets larger, the binomial distribution becomes increasingly negatively skewed
• when p = 0.5 (i.e. the two possible outcomes are equally likely to happen), the binomial distribution is symmetrical
• for large sample sizes, the binomial distribution can often be approximated to a Normal distribution with mean = np and variance = np(1-p) [see section 5.3 for further details].

5.2 Poisson distribution

Many discrete continuous measures arise from counting the number of events which occur:
• in a fixed time interval (e.g. epileptic fits experienced by a patient in a year)

- in a fixed space (e.g. numbers of cells in a graticule on a microscope field/slide).

Such measures have a theoretical Poisson distribution. This is characterised by the mean number of events; the variance of a Poisson distribution is equal to the mean.

5.3 Normal/Gaussian distribution

MANY CONTINUOUS BIOLOGICAL MEASURES APPROXIMATE CLOSELY TO A MATHEMATICAL ENTITY CALLED THE **NORMAL** OR **GAUSSIAN** DISTRIBUTION

Such observations have a frequency distribution which is characterised by being 'bell-shaped' (unimodal) and symmetrical about its central value (Fig. 7).

For a Normal distribution:
- the distribution is completely defined by its mean and standard deviation

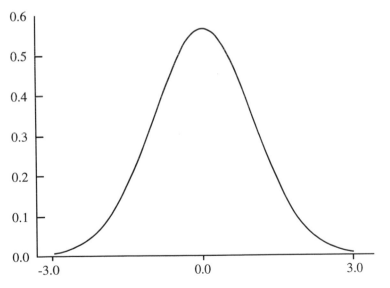

Fig. 7: The (standard) Normal/Gaussian distribution

- **mean = median = mode**
- quantiles are usually computed by inserting values for the mean and standard deviation in the formula for the Normal distribution.

The frequency curve for a Normal distribution can be used to determine the proportion of observations lying (theoretically) within a stated range. For example (Fig. 8):

- 68.2% (approximately two-thirds) of the observations lie within one standard deviation either side of the mean
- 95% of the observations lie within 1.96 standard deviations either side of the mean
- 95.5% (i.e. fractionally over 95%) of the observations lie within 2 standard deviations either side of the mean (i.e. less than 5% of the observations lie further than 2 standard deviations away from the mean)
- 99.8% (virtually all) of the observations lie within 3 standard deviations of the mean.

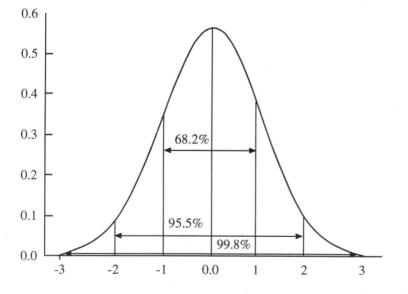

Fig. 8: The (standard) Normal/Gaussian distribution: proportions of observations between 1, 2 and 3 standard deviations of mean value

For large sample sizes:
- the binomial distribution approximates to a Normal distribution with mean = np and variance = np(1-p) (see also section 5.1)
- the Poisson distribution approximates to a Normal distribution with mean = variance (see also section 5.2).

Any data (X) with a Normal distribution can be converted into the **standard Normal distribution** (Z) by subtracting the mean from each observation and then dividing by the standard deviation:

$$Z = (X - \text{mean})/\text{standard deviation}$$

These Z values always have a *standard Normal distribution* which has a mean of zero and a standard deviation of one. Thus, tables which detail the standard Normal distribution can, in fact, be used for data with any Normal distribution.

Data which have a statistically Normal distribution are not necessarily normal in the ordinary (clinical) sense of this word:
- haemoglobin levels may follow a statistically Normal distribution, but a value of 8 mg/dl would be clinically abnormal, indicating the presence of a disease state
- resting pulse rates may follow a statistically non-Normal distribution, but a value of 72 beats/minute would be clinically normal.

5.4 Non-Normal continuous distributions

Many other biological variables follow distributions which are unimodal but are not symmetrical. These are called *skew distributions*.
A distribution which has:
- a long tail on the right (i.e. a tendency to large values) is *positively skewed* (Fig. 9a)
- a long tail on the left (i.e. a tendency to small values) is *negatively skewed* (Fig. 9b).

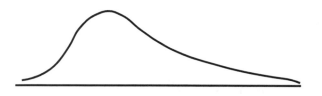

Fig. 9a: Positively skewed, continuous distribution

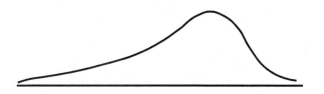

Fig. 9b: Negatively skewed, continuous distribution

- For variables which are skewed (non-Normal): **mean ≠ median ≠ mode**
- if the variable is *positively skewed*: **mean > median > mode**
- if the variable is *negatively skewed*: **mean < median < mode**.

Positively and negatively skewed distributions are effectively mirror images about the mode. Moving from the mode (the apex of the frequency distribution) into the long tail produces the relationship:
mode → median → mean (Fig. 10).

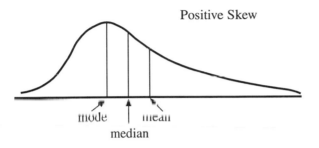

Positive Skew

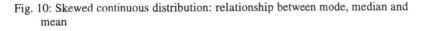

Fig. 10: Skewed continuous distribution: relationship between mode, median and mean

For a non-Normal distribution, quantiles are usually computed directly from the data (observations).

Many naturally skewed/'non-Normal' distributions can be **transformed into** Normal distributions. Some such distributions which occur frequently in biological systems are:

• the *log-Normal* distribution (one of the most common types of positively skewed data, this can be transformed into a Normal distribution by taking the (natural) logarithm of each observation)

• the distribution of data such as counts or the number of times an event occurs in a fixed time period is often only moderately positively skewed; this can be transformed to a Normal distribution by taking the square root of each observation

• the distribution of data such as survival times is often extremely positively skewed, requiring the reciprocal transformation (1/observation) to obtain a Normal distribution

• the distribution of proportions (percentages) can be skewed if the observations extend to 0 and/or 1 (100%); this can sometimes be converted into a Normal distribution by using one of several complex mathematical transformations (e.g. arcsine, probit, logit).

Complex statistical tests exist which determine the most appropriate (Normalising) transformation for a set of data and measure its success. Statistical analysis methods appropriate for Normally distributed data are used on the transformed values; the results can, under certain circumstances, be **detransformed** back into their original units at the end of the analysis.

6: CONFIDENCE INTERVALS

6.1 Standard errors

6.1.1 Quantitative data

A sample of 250 individuals selected at random from the general population of hypertensive patients were treated with a drug which reduces blood pressure. If changes in diastolic blood pressure follow a Normal distribution:
- the mean change experienced by this sample will provide an estimate of the therapeutic efficacy of the drug
- successive samples of 250 individuals selected randomly from the same population and treated in the same way will provide additional estimates of the drug's therapeutic effect
- the estimates obtained will all be similar but not necessarily equal.

The distribution of these means is called the **sampling distribution** of the sample means.

If the individual observations follow a Normal distribution with mean μ and variance σ^2, the means of a series of random samples of size n will also follow a Normal distribution with mean μ but much smaller variance (σ^2/n).

> The standard deviation of the sampling distribution is called the **standard error of the sample mean (SEM)**.
> $$SEM = \sigma/\sqrt{n}$$
> = standard deviation of the individual observations divided by the square root of the number of observations in the sample.

In practice, the population variance is usually unknown, so has to be estimated from the study sample. For a random sample of size n:
- the sample variance is s^2, computed as described in section 4.2.2
- the sample standard deviation is s
- the sample standard error (SEM) is $s/\sqrt{n}$.

As the size of the sample (n) increases, the standard error becomes increasingly small. If a sufficiently large sample could be taken:
- the sample mean would be a very close estimate of the true population mean
- the sample standard deviation would be a very close estimate of the true population standard deviation
- the standard error would approach close to zero!

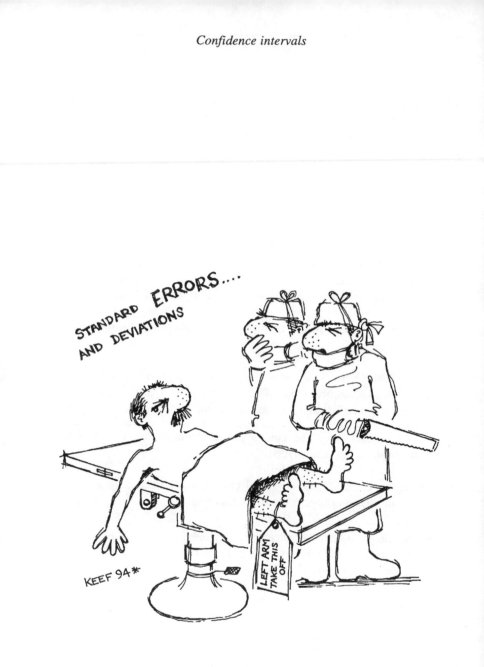

The SEM provides a <u>measure of the spread of the sample means</u> about the (unknown) true population mean (and must not be confused with the standard deviation, which provides a measure of how much individual observations are spread around the true population mean).

The SEM is often used to determine how close to the true population mean the sample mean is likely to be (this process is described in detail in section 6.3).

6.1.2 Qualitative data

As in section 6.1.1 above, successive samples of 250 individuals selected at random from the general population of hypertensive patients were treated with a drug which reduces blood pressure. The proportion of patients in each sample who experienced a mild unwanted side-effect provide a set of estimates of the (mild) toxicity incidence level associated with the drug. Again, the estimates will all be similar but not necessarily equal.

In a sample of n individuals, if the number falling into a particular category (e.g. who experience a side-effect) is r, the proportion falling into this category is $r/n = p$.

For small samples, the sampling distribution of p can be determined exactly using the properties of the binomial distribution (see also section 5.1).

For large samples, the extent to which the observed proportions (p) spread around the true population proportion is determined using the Normal approximation to the binomial distribution (see section 5.1). It can be shown that, in this situation:
- variance of $p = p \cdot (1-p)/n$
- standard error of $p = \sqrt{[p \cdot (1-p)/n]}$.

6.2 Student t-distribution

The properties of samples drawn from a Normal distribution (section 6.1.1) hold for large samples. However, if the sample size is small (≤ 60):
- the population variance will tend to be under-estimated
- the sample means, when converted to a standard Normal distribution (section 5.3), follow a distribution which is symmetrical but has much longer tails (i.e. has much greater spread) than a Normal distribution.

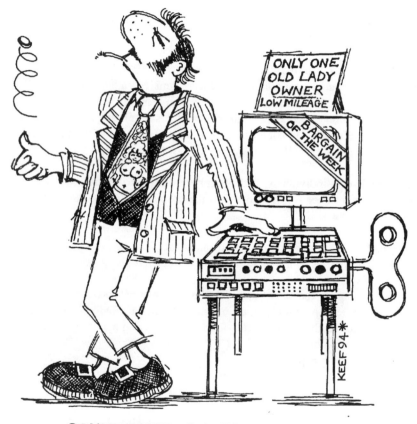

CONFIDENCE LIMITS ......

The exact mathematical form of the sampling distribution for small samples drawn from a Normal distribution was published in 1908 by W. S. Gossett. Because his employers (the Guinness brewery in Dublin) would not allow him to publish, Gossett submitted his paper under the pseudonym 'Student'. As a consequence, the distribution has become known universally as the **Student t-distribution.**

The precise shape (degree of spread) of the Student t-distribution depends on the number of degrees of freedom for the variance estimate (section 4.2.2). For a single sample mean:

degrees of freedom = n − 1 (number of observations in the sample minus 1)

As the sample size increases:
- the degrees of freedom increase
- the more closely the t-distribution resembles the standard Normal distribution
- for samples in excess of 60 observations, the Student t-distribution is virtually indistinguishable from the standard Normal distribution.

When computing confidence limits (section 6.3) or significance tests (chapter 7):
- the standard Normal distribution is not appropriate for small samples so the Student t-distribution <u>must</u> be used
- the standard Normal distribution <u>is</u> appropriate for large samples, but so is the Student t-distribution as the two are indistinguishable.

FOR PRACTICAL PURPOSES, THEREFORE, THE STUDENT
t-DISTRIBUTION TENDS TO BE USED FOR ALL SAMPLES

6.3 Confidence limits

In a random sample of patients selected for a clinical trial of a new hypertensive drug:
- the mean change in diastolic blood pressure will provide an estimate of the true (average) effect of the drug
- the proportion of patients who experience an unwanted mild side-effect will provide an estimate of the true (average) toxicity incidence level of the drug.

A properly selected random sample will:
* be representative of the study population
* produce estimates very close to, but not necessarily equal to, the true population value.

True population values are not known (if they were, the clinical trial would not be needed!).

A *confidence interval*:
* is computed from the sample standard error
* provides a measure of the extent to which a sample estimate is likely to differ from the true population value (i.e. a measure of the degree of precision/uncertainty associated with the sample estimate)
* indicates, with a stated level of certainty (e.g. 95%), the range of values within which the true population mean is likely to lie.

6.3.1 Confidence intervals for a Normal distribution (quantitative data)

For a continuous measure with a Normal distribution, the α% confidence interval for the population mean μ is given by :

$$M - (t . SEM) < \mu < M + (t . SEM)$$

or, more conventionally, by

$$M \pm (t . SEM)$$

where M is the mean and SEM is the standard error of random sample of size n; the multiplication term t is the $(1 - \alpha)$% value of the Student t-distribution corresponding to (n-1) degrees of freedom (for large samples, the value of t can be replaced by the equivalent percentage point on the standard Normal distribution).

* *It can be stated with α% certainty that the true population mean lies within the α% confidence interval.*

The most frequently reported confidence interval is the **95% *confidence interval.*** It can be stated with 95% certainty that the population mean lies within this interval.

For large samples, the value of t is 1.96, making the formula:

$$M \pm (1.96 . SEM)$$

In practice, *approximate 95% confidence intervals* are sufficient, obtained by rounding the multiplication factor (t) to a more easily computed value of 2:

$$M \pm (2 . SEM)$$

Confidence intervals do not have to be 95% certain of including the population mean. The desired level of confidence can be increased or decreased, which in turn increases or decreases respectively the size of the interval. Thus, for large samples:

99% confidence limits are defined by: $M \pm (2.58 . SEM)$

90% confidence limits are defined by: $M \pm (1.65 . SEM)$

For a given level of confidence:
- a narrow interval indicates that the sample estimate has good (high) precision
- a wide interval indicates that the sample estimate has poor (low) precision.

Confidence intervals become increasingly narrow (the precision of the sample estimate becomes increasingly better) as:
- the sample size increases (this reduces the value of the standard error)
- the variability of the data decreases (this also reduces the value of the standard error)
- the degree of confidence required for the population mean decreases (this reduces the value of the multiplication factor t).

Confidence intervals can also be computed for differences between means; these indicate the likely extremes for the true difference between the means (i.e. the true difference in the efficacies of the treatments being compared).

6.3.2 Confidence intervals for a binomial distribution (qualitative data)

For a categorical (qualitative) measure, the α% confidence interval for the proportion of patients in a sample of size n with a particular characteristic is computed:

- **for small samples**: exactly from the properties of the binomial distribution (see also section 5.1) – extensive tables exist for these (e.g. Documenta Geigy)
- **for large samples**: using the approximation of the binomial distribution to the Normal distribution (see also section 5.1) – if $\hat{p}$ is the estimate from a sample of size n of the true proportion **p** of the population with a specific characteristic, the $\alpha\%$ confidence limits for **p** is given by:

$$\hat{p} \pm (t \cdot \sqrt{[\hat{p} \cdot (1-\hat{p})/n]}$$

6.4 Confidence limits for individual observations (reference ranges)

By using standard errors in the computation of confidence limits, statements can be made about the likely range of values within which a population value such as a mean or proportion lies.

In many clinical situations, it is more important to know the range of values within which the observation from an individual patient is likely to lie.

Such intervals are called *reference/normal ranges*. These are computed using the same formulae as in section 6.3, but **with the standard error replaced by the standard deviation.**

7.1 Basic principles

A simple clinical trial was carried out on a group of patients to compare the reductions in blood pressure produced by two drugs. Even if the drugs had identical therapeutic effects, it is unlikely that the observed mean changes in blood pressure would be exactly the same. Thus, if a numerical difference <u>was</u> observed between the estimated effects of the two drugs:

- was it the result of chance (random variation), or
- was it due to a real difference in their therapeutic effects (systematic variation)?

Significance tests are statistical methods which allow a choice to be made between these two conclusions using data obtained from a suitably designed study. This is done by setting up and comparing two hypotheses:

- **Null hypothesis** – central to significance testing and usually a statement of 'no difference'
  e.g. the <u>true</u> therapeutic effects of the two drugs were identical/the <u>true</u> difference in the mean changes in blood pressure produced by the two drugs was zero.
- **Alternative hypothesis** – usually a statement of 'real difference' taking one of two forms:
  - *Two-sided* – the direction of the difference <u>is not</u> stated in advance
    e.g. the <u>true</u> therapeutic effects of the two drugs were <u>not</u> identical/the <u>true</u> difference in the mean blood pressure changes produced by the drugs was <u>not</u> zero/drug A could have a lesser or greater therapeutic effect than drug B
  - *One-sided* – the direction of the difference <u>is</u> stated in advance
    e.g. the true therapeutic effect of drug A was greater than that of drug B/the change in blood pressure produced by A was really greater than that produced by B.

All of the significance tests described in this chapter (including those defined as 'non-parametric') can be computed for either a one-sided or a two-sided alternative hypothesis.

On completion of the study, appropriate significance tests are selected (see sections 6.3, 6.4 and 6.5). When computed, these provide a **test statistic** for each of the study measures (variables). Each test statistic is converted into a **p-value**.

SIGNIFICANCE TESTING

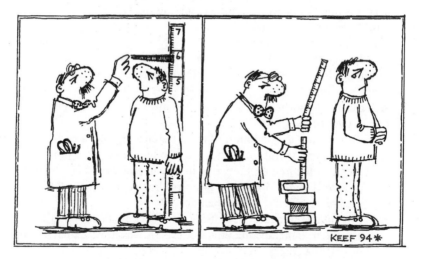

A **p-value** is an estimate of the probability that the difference observed in the study (or one more extreme) could have occurred if the Null hypothesis is true. A p-value can be thought of as the probability that the observed difference could have occurred by chance.

Clearly, as a p-value becomes smaller, the difference observed becomes less and less consistent with the Null hypothesis. Eventually, a point is reached where the p value becomes so small that the decision has to be taken that the study data can no longer be accepted as supporting the Null hypothesis.

The value of p at which this decision is taken is called the **significance level** (or **critical level**) When p falls below this level:
* the observed difference is so unlikely to have occurred by chance that the Null hypothesis must be rejected and the Alternative hypothesis (of a real difference) accepted
* the difference observed between the drugs is defined as being **statistically significant**.

The choice of level for a significance level is largely artificial; increasingly, the actual p-value obtained is produced by all good statistical computer packages. Conventionally, however, statistical significance is usually set at 5% (1 in 20).

Setting the critical level of p as low as 5% may seem extreme. The testing of hypotheses, however, is analogous to the process of trial by jury. Jurors are directed by a judge to return a guilty verdict only if the weight of evidence is against the defendant; similarly, researchers are required to reject the Null hypothesis of no difference only if the weight of evidence (*the balance of probabilities*) from the clinical study is overwhelmingly against it.

Significance tests are prone to two types of error, i.e. there are two situations in which the p-value can lead to an erroneous conclusion:

Types of error possible with test statistics	True situation	
	Null hypothesis true	Null hypothesis false
Conclusion Null hypothesis true from test	Correct	Type II error
statistic : Null hypothesis false	Type I error	Correct

- A **Type I error** (false-positive result) occurs if the Null hypothesis is rejected when it is actually true (the effects of the drugs are interpreted as being different when they are not). The probability of committing a Type I error, often denoted by the Greek letter α, is equal to the significance level (i.e. is equal to the p-value).
  With a conventional 5% significance level, a significant difference will occur purely by chance once in every 20 tests performed on average (even though no difference exists).
  One way of minimising the risk of a Type I error is to reject the Null hypothesis only if the p-value is extremely low (e.g. $p \leq 0.001$, or even $p \leq 0.0001$).
- A **Type II error** (false-negative result) occurs if the Null hypothesis is accepted when it is actually false (the effects of the drugs are interpreted as being equal when they are actually different). The probability of committing a Type II error is often denoted by the Greek letter ß.
- The **power** of a study is defined as the probability that a Type II error will <u>not</u> be made. In mathematical terms, the power of a study = $1 - ß$.
  Suppose a difference (of pre-stated size) truly exists between the effects of two drugs. A comparative clinical trial is to be carried out to detect this difference. The power is the probability that, when the study is completed and the data obtained is analysed, a statistically significant difference will be detected.

7.2 Clinical vs statistical significance

Clinical significance is:
- the smallest therapeutic effect for a drug which is clinically valuable, or
- the smallest difference between the therapeutic effects of two drugs which is clinically important.

The magnitude and clinical importance of any effect found to be statistically significant in a clinical trial must be taken into account when interpreting the result. A superior pharmacological effect may be found for drug A than for drug B, but if the side-effect profile or tolerability for drug A is very poor, it may actually be clinically inferior to drug B.

A small therapeutic effect of a drug may emerge as statistically significant but may be clinically unimportant. **Statistical significance is not the same as clinical significance.**

A clinically significant difference may exist, but the study may not have been sufficiently powerful to detect it. A statistically non-significant difference, irrespective of its numerical size, has an unacceptably high probability of occurring by chance and cannot be interpreted as clinically significant. **The absence of statistical significance gives no information regarding clinical significance.**

> STATISTICAL SIGNIFICANCE DOES NOT IMPLY
> CLINICAL SIGNIFICANCE

7.3 Estimation of sample size

The design of a clinical study to compare the effects of two (or more) treatments must ensure that, as far as possible, the risks of Type I and Type II errors are minimised. This is achieved by considering the following mathematically inter-related factors:

* the acceptable level for the Type I error rate (conventionally, this is usually set at 5%)
* the acceptable level for the Type II error rate (conventionally, this is usually set at either 10% or 20%, corresponding to power levels of 90% and 80% respectively)
* the difference between the effects of the treatments defined as being clinically significant
* the level of the variation inherent to the study's primary (main) outcome measure (*experimental error*).

All of these factors affect the number of patients which must be recruited to the study (*sample size*). Reducing the Type I error rate, the Type II error rate and/or the size of the difference in treatment effects defined as clinically significant, increases the number of patients required, as does increasing the size of the experimental error associated with the outcome measure. Formulae exist which determine the relationship between these measures and sample size for most experimental situations. Increasingly, summaries of these calculations are being demanded in reports of study reports submitted to medical journals/conferences.

7.4 General form of test statistics

Many test statistics are derived either from data which can be assumed to have a Normal distribution or (for large sample sizes) can be approximated to a Normal distribution. The **primary summary statistic** (e.g. the mean difference between the effects of two treatments, or the proportion of patients responding to a treatment) will also have a Normal distribution.

Under the constraint of the Null hypothesis, this Normal distribution will have:
* a mean equal to a hypothesised value (usually zero when evaluating differences)
* a known or estimated variance.

The primary statistic is transformed into a test statistic with a standard Normal distribution by subtracting the (hypothesised) mean and dividing by its standard error (section 5.3). This produces a test statistic with one of the following general forms:
* Test statistic = mean difference/standard error of difference
* Test statistic = (estimated statistic – hypothesised value)/standard error of estimate.

Test statistics have no real intuitive value in their own right. They provide a means to an end, being required as a transition stage in obtaining an estimate of the p-value.

7.5 Significance tests for qualitative data

Two treatments for stomach cancer were compared in a clinical trial using different groups of patients. This produced the following estimates of the cure rates for each treatment:
* n_A patients were treated with drug A and n_B patients were treated with drug B
* a patients were cured by drug A and b patients were cured by drug B
* $(n_A - a)$ patients were not cured by drug A and $(n_B - b)$ patients were not cured by drug B
* estimated cure rates: drug $A = \hat{p}_A = a / n_A$
  drug $B = \hat{p}_B = b / n_B$

Both cure rates are proportions which follow theoretical binomial distributions (section 5.1). If the conventional Null hypothesis is true, the cure rates of the two treatments are identical, so the results for the two drugs can be combined to obtain the best available estimate of:

- the common cure rate $\hat{p} = (n_A \cdot \hat{p}_A + n_B \cdot \hat{p}_B)/(n_A + n_B)$
  $$= (a + b)/(n_A + n_B)$$
- the common non-cure rate $\hat{q} = 1 - \hat{p}$.

The significance of the difference between the cure rates can be determined in two ways.

7.5.1 Using the binomial distribution

For small samples ($n \le 30$), the probability that the observed difference (or one more extreme) could have occurred under the Null hypothesis can be computed exactly from the properties of the binomial distribution. This is known as the *Fisher exact test*. It is computationally complex and cannot be used for large samples.

For large samples ($n > 30$), the binomial distribution approximates to a Normal distribution for which:

- mean difference in cure rates = $\hat{p}_A - \hat{p}_B$
- standard error of difference in cure rates = se($\hat{p}$)
  $$= \sqrt{[(\hat{p} \cdot \hat{q} / n_A) + (\hat{p} \cdot \hat{q} / n_B)]}$$

Thus, the following test statistic has a standard Normal distribution:

> z = (mean difference in cure rates)/(standard error of difference in cure rates)

The p-value for the difference in cure rates can be obtained by referring the value of z to tables of the standard Normal distribution.

7.5.2 Using the chi-squared (χ^2) test/contingency tables

The results of the comparative study of two treatments for stomach cancer can be summarised in general terms in the form of a 2 x 2 contingency table:

Outcome	Treatment A	Treatment B	Total
Cured	a	b	a + b
Not cured	c $(n_A - a)$	d $(n_B - b)$	c + d
Total	a + c (n_A)	b + d (n_B)	a + b + c + d $(n_A + n_B)$

For this contingency table:
- the values a, b, c and d are the **observed values** for the cells in the contingency table
- the probability of 'cure' on drug A is estimated by $\hat{p}_A = a/(a + c) = a/n_A$
- the probability of 'cure' on drug B is estimated by $\hat{p}_B = b/(b + d) = b/n_B$
- the common cure rate under the conventional Null hypothesis that the cure rates of the two treatments are identical:
  $\hat{p} = (a + b)/(n_A + n_B) = (a + b)/(a + b + c + d)$

Using the best estimate ($\hat{p}$) of the common cure rate, the **expected values** for each cell in the contingency table can be computed. For example, for treatment group A:
- the number of patients treated was (a + c)
- the <u>proportion</u> expected to be cured (under the Null hypothesis) was $\hat{p}$
- the <u>number</u> expected to be cured is $\hat{p}. (a + c)$.

The expected values for the remaining contingency table cells can be computed similarly.

The test statistic for the contingency table is obtained by computing for each cell the statistic:

(observed value – expected value)²/expected value

and then summing the values obtained over all of the cells in the table. The test statistic produced has a theoretical χ^2-distribution.

The p-value is obtained by referring the test statistic to tables of the χ^2-distribution with appropriate degrees of freedom. The degrees of freedom for a contingency table χ^2 statistic are equal to:

(number of rows in table – 1) x (number of columns in table -1)

Computationally, the χ^2 test statistic is equivalent to that produced in section 7.5.1 and can be used for any size of contingency table. It is based on a number of approximations, so should only be used when the Fisher exact test cannot be computed.

Several very important criteria restrict the validity of this test:

• the approximations are most likely to break down for a 2 (rows) x 2 (columns) contingency table – the degree of fit is improved by applying Yates' continuity correction – this correction should always be applied for a 2 x 2 table, but is not required for larger tables

• the approximations also tend to break down if the expected cell frequencies are small – strictly, the test is valid only if all expected cell frequencies exceed 5   however, a more relaxed rule is often advocated, which requires 80% of the expected cell frequencies to exceed 5 and all of them to exceed 1

• contingency table analyses are valid only if a, b, c and d are actual numbers of patients; converting the numbers to percentages totally invalidates the test statistic.

7.6 Significance tests for quantitative (continuous) data

7.6.1 Parametric and nonparametric methods

When a continuous variable can be assumed to follow a Normal distribution:

• parametric statistical methods are appropriate to evaluate the difference in the therapeutic effects of two (or more) study groups

• the appropriate summary statistics which should be used are means and standard deviations/standard errors.

When a continuous variable cannot be assumed to follow a Normal distribution:

• attempts should be made to transform the data into a Normal distribution (section 5.4)

• if a Normalising transformation cannot be found, and the data do not follow any other recognisable distribution, nonparametric/distribution-free statistical methods are appropriate to evaluate the difference in the therapeutic effects of two (or more) study groups

• as their name suggests, nonparametric/distribution-free methods make no assumption about the nature of the underlying data distribution

• the appropriate summary statistics which should be used are medians and ranges

- many nonparametric methods involve ranking the data into ascending order and replacing the original observations with their ranks – the test statistics are computed using these rank values.

7.6.2 Independent samples

Observations collected from two distinct groups of individuals constitute *independent samples*.

In a simple clinical trial, blood glucose levels were measured in two groups of individuals; the n_1 subjects in group 1 had a normal diet, while the n_2 subjects in group 2 had a diet with a high sugar content.

If the blood glucose levels can be assumed to follow a Normal distribution:
- the *Student independent samples/unpaired t-test* is used to evaluate the difference between the mean blood glucose levels of the two groups
- under the Null hypothesis that the means are equal, the test statistic takes the form:
  (mean for group 1 – mean for group 2)/standard error of difference
- this test statistic has a Student t-distribution with $n_1 + n_2 - 2$ degrees of freedom (i.e. the total number of observations minus the number of mean values calculated)
- if the variances of the two samples are equal[†], the test is straightforward (a pooled estimate of the common variance is used to compute the test statistic)
- if the variances are <u>not</u> equal, the test is invalid (however, an approximate method can be computed using separate variance estimates from the two samples).

If the blood glucose levels cannot be assumed to follow a Normal distribution:
- the *Mann-Whitney U-test* is used to compare the distributions of blood glucose levels in the two study groups
- this test is the nonparametric equivalent of the Student independent samples/unpaired t-test
- for small samples, tables exist which convert the test statistic U into the

† The equality of the sample variances can be tested as follows:
- compute the variance estimates (s_1^2 and s_2^2) of the two samples
- compute the ratio of the larger variance estimate (s_1^2) to the smaller variance estimate (s_2^2)
- this ratio (s_1^2/s_2^2) has an F-distribution with $(n_1 -1)$ and (n_2-1) degrees of freedom.

probability that the observed difference (or one more extreme) could have arisen if the Null hypothesis of no difference between the two groups was true (p-value)
- for large samples, U is converted into a test statistic with a Standard Normal distribution, from which the p-value can be determined by reference to tables.

7.6.3 Dependent samples

Observations collected from the same group of individuals on two separate occasions (a within-group comparison) constitute **dependent/paired samples.**

Blood glucose levels were measured in a group of n individuals before and after a meal with a high sugar content.

If the blood glucose levels can be assumed to follow a Normal distribution:
- the *Student dependent samples/paired t-test* is used to evaluate the difference between the mean blood glucose levels on the two occasions
- the test statistic is obtained by computing the difference between the two blood levels for each individual separately and then calculating the mean of these differences
- the test statistic under the Null hypothesis that the means are equal takes the form:
  mean difference/standard error of difference
- this test statistic has a Student t-distribution with n 1 (the total number of pairs of observations minus one) degrees of freedom.

If the blood glucose levels cannot be assumed to follow a Normal distribution:
- the *Wilcoxon matched-pairs rank-sum test* is used to compare the distributions of the mean blood glucose levels on the two occasions
- this test is the nonparametric equivalent of the Student dependent samples t-test
- for small samples, tables exist which convert the test statistic T into the probability that the observed difference (or one more extreme) could have arisen if the Null hypothesis of no difference between the two occasions was true (p-value)
- for large samples, T is converted into a test statistic with a Standard Normal distribution, from which the p-value can be determined by reference to tables.

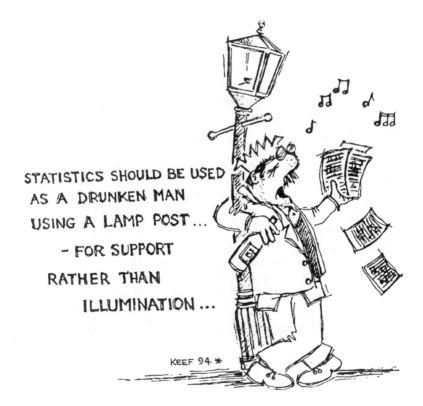

7.7 Significance tests vs confidence limits

Confidence limits and significance tests examine different aspects of the same question so are very closely related. For example, if a continuous variable has a Normal distribution, the formulae for confidence intervals are the same as for the corresponding Student t-test.

In general terms, confidence limits are more informative than significance tests. This is particularly true in situations where a difference is not statistically significant. Confidence intervals provide information about whether or not a 'real' difference exists between two treatments, but then also quantifies the likely size of any difference.

Example
The difference in the mean blood glucose levels of two groups of people with normal and high sugar content diets was 2.3 mmol/l:
a)   the 95% confidence interval for this difference was +0.7 to +3.9 mmol/l: as this interval does not includes the value 0 (zero), the difference between the two groups can be interpreted as being significant (i.e. the Null hypothesis of no difference between the groups must be *rejected*) – in addition, we can say with 95% certainty that mean glucose levels are between 0.7 mmol/l and 3.9 mmol/l higher on average in people with a high sugar diet compared with those with a normal diet
b)   the 95% confidence interval for this difference was -0.7 to +5.3 mmol/l: this interval includes the value 0, so the difference between the two groups can be interpreted as being non-significant (i.e. the Null hypothesis of no difference between the groups must be *accepted*) – in addition, we can say with 95% certainty that blood glucose levels could be as much as 0.7 mmol/l higher on average people with a normal diet or as much as 5.3 mmol/l higher on average in people with a high sugar diet.

The confidence interval for an individual group quantifies the likely range of responses for that group, but cannot be used directly for comparisons with other groups. When evaluating the difference between the efficacies of two treatments, the degree of overlap of the confidence limits for each treatment mean cannot be used to determine whether the difference is statistically significant. This can only be determined by computing the (95%) confidence limits for the actual difference in the means.
The results of an experiment should ideally be presented using confidence

intervals. The corresponding test statistics and their p-values can be reported also, but this is tantamount to tautology.

8: MEASURES OF ASSOCIATION

8.1 Scatterplots

The most effective initial way of assessing whether or not there is an association between two variables is graphically. This is best achieved by constructing a **scatterplot**, in which:

- the variable plotted on the vertical axis is called the **dependent** (y) variable
- the variable plotted on the horizontal axis is called the **independent** (x) variable.

x and y are sometimes referred to as the **predictor** and **predicted** variables respectively; conventionally, values of y are estimated (predicted) for known values of the x variable.

<u>Example</u>
Levels of anxiety (x) and depression (y) were measured in a group of 15 patients with diabetes. The most effective initial way of assessing whether or not there is an association between the two symptoms is to construct a scatterplot (Fig. 11). This shows a definite but weak relationship, with anxiety levels tending to be slightly greater than average depression levels.

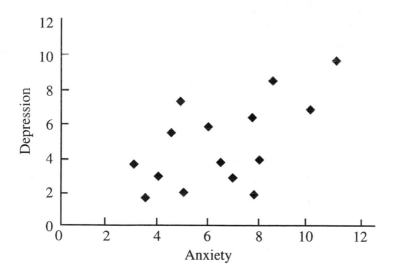

Fig. 11: Scatter plot suggesting an association between anxiety and depression

8.2 Correlation

Individuals with a high dietary salt intake appear to have higher blood pressure levels than those with a low intake. A clinical trial was carried out in which the two characteristics were measured in a group of individuals drawn at random from the general population.

If a scatterplot of the two characteristics suggests that they may be (mathematically) related, a **correlation coefficient** can be computed to estimate the **strength of the association** between the two characteristics (variables) to be estimated.

8.2.1 Pearson correlation coefficient

The Pearson correlation coefficient measures the strength of the relationship between two variables when:
- both variables are continuous
- at least one of the variables follows a Normal distribution
- the relationship is <u>linear</u> (i.e. the Pearson correlation coefficient measures how close the relationship between the observations is to a straight line).

The Pearson correlation coefficient is usually denoted by the letter **r**.

The correlation coefficient has a number of important properties:
- r only takes values in the range -1 to +1 inclusive
- a value of r greater than zero implies a *positive relationship* between the two variables (as one variable increases, the other increases also).
- a value for r less than zero implies a *negative relationship* between the two variables (as one variable increases, the other decreases)
- if $r = +1$ or $r = -1$, the two variables are perfectly correlated and all of the observations lie on a straight line (both relationships represented in Fig. 12 have a correlation exactly equal to +1).

As the value of r approaches zero, the association between the two variables becomes weaker, manifested by an increasing scatter of the points about the line of perfect relationship (Fig. 13).

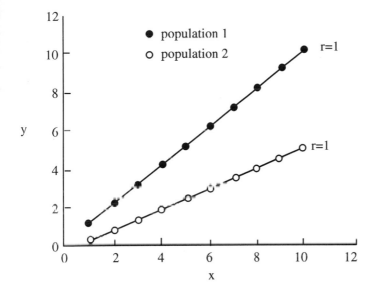

Fig. 12: Perfect positive correlations

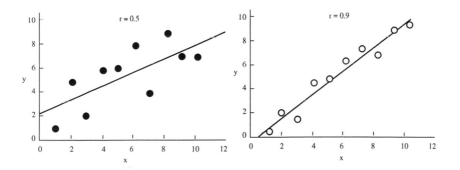

Fig. 13: Positive correlations

- when r = 0, there is no linear association between the two variables (the values of one variable are not linearly related)
- the correlation between two measures is often regarded as *strong* if r < -0.5 or r > +0.5
- the correlation between two measures is often regarded as *weak* if -0.5 ≤ r ≤ +0.5
- r is a dimensionless statistic (i.e. has no units) and is independent of the units of the two variables being evaluated
- r does not allow the value of one variable to be estimated from the value of the other (r measures how closely the observations conform to a linear relationship but provides no information about the form of that straight line)
- although r measures the strength of a linear relationship, the value of r is not equal to the slope of the line.

8.2.2 Spearman correlation coefficient

If an examination of the scattergram suggests that the relationship between the variables is not linear, or if the relationship is linear but the conditions required by the Pearson correlation coefficient do not apply, it may be possible to use the **Spearman correlation coefficient** instead.

The Spearman correlation coefficient also measures the strength of the relationship between two variables. It requires:
- both variables to be continuous or ordered categories
- no assumption to be made about the distribution of either variable
- the relationship between the two variables to be merely monotonic (i.e. an increase in one variable is associated always with an increase or always with a decrease in the other variable – Fig. 14).

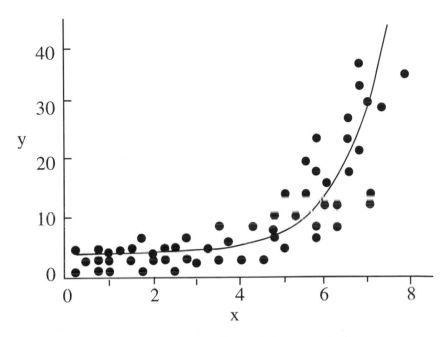

Fig. 14: Non-linear (curvilinear) monotonic correlation

The Spearman correlation coefficient has the same mathematical properties as the Pearson correlation coefficient (section 8.2.1).

The Pearson correlation coefficient is computed using the actual observation values; the Spearman correlation coefficient is computed using the identical mathematical formula, but using the ranks of the observation values for each variable.

The Spearman correlation coefficient is the nonparametric equivalent of the Pearson correlation coefficient.

8.2.3 Complex non-linear relationships

If the relationship between two variables has at least one clear turning point (i.e. it changes direction at least once – Fig. 15), neither of the correlation coefficients described above is valid. Although there may be an obvious association between the variables, both coefficients will be (close to) zero. More complex mathematical methods, outside the scope of this book, are required to assess the strength of such relationships.

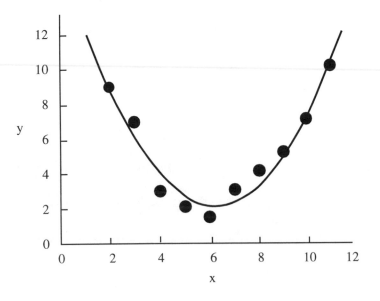

Fig. 15: Non-linear non-monotonic correlation

8.2.4 Significance/confidence limits for correlations

The correlation coefficient has a non-standard distribution. However, the **Fisher z-transformation** enables r to be converted into a standard Normal distribution, from which:
- confidence limits can be estimated for r
- the Null hypothesis that r = 0 (i.e. there is no association between the two variables) can be tested.

Caution should be exercised when interpreting the significance of a correlation. The p-value obtained is dependent both on the strength of the association and, in a sense more importantly, on the sample size. Thus:
- a small correlation can be statistically significant if the sample size is very large
- a large correlation can be statistically non-significant if the sample size is small.

A more useful statistic is the square of the correlation coefficient (usually denoted by R^2). This is the proportion of the variation in one of the variables accounted for by its relationship with the other, and can often put r into a more realistic context; e.g. if a correlation coefficient of 0.3 is statistically significant, only $(0.3)^2 = 0.09 = 9\%$ of the variation in either variable is accounted for, suggesting that the association may be of little clinical value.

A strong correlation does not give any information about the size of any effect. Association and causality are discussed in detail in Chapter 9. However, it is worth emphasising here that a significant correlation between two variables does not imply that they are causally related.

8.3 Linear regression

If a straight line relationship is established between two variables, **linear regression methods** can be used to determine the exact mathematical form of the relationship. From this, predictions can be made about one of the variables from the values of the other variable.

Linear regression is a statistical method for estimating the equation of the straight line which best describes the relationship between two variables x and y (Fig. 16). The line takes the form

$$y = a + b.x$$

- y is called the **dependent variable**
- x is called the **independent variable**
- a is called the **intercept** (and is equal to the value of y when x = 0)
- b is called the **regression coefficient/slope of the regression line** (and is a measure of the rate at which y changes for unit increases in the value of x).

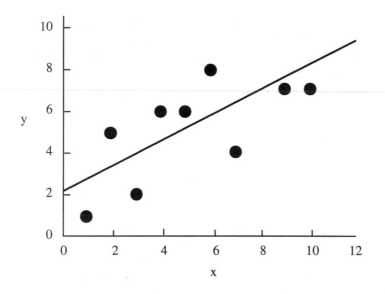

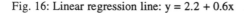

Fig. 16: Linear regression line: y = 2.2 + 0.6x

A regression equation can be used to predict the value of the dependent variable (y) for a known value of the independent variable (x). This should be done only within the range of values for which the dependent variable has been tested (**interpolation**); estimating values outside this range (**extrapolation**) produces estimates of y which become increasingly unreliable. Predicted values of y should always be presented with their 95% confidence limit.

Confidence limits can be estimated for both a and b. Tests of the hypotheses a = 0 and b = 0 can be constructed. The statistical test for the slope of the regression line is mathematically equivalent to the test of significance for the correlation r between the variables.

If the relationship between the variables is non-linear, a transformation of one or both variables can often produce a linear relationship (e.g. if two variables are exponentially related, taking the natural logarithms of one variable produces a linear relationship). If this is not possible, **non-linear regression methods** must be used. These methods are outside the scope of this book.

If the relationship between the dependent variable and several independent variables is of interest, **multiple linear regression methods** can be employed. This produces a mathematical relationship from which the value of the dependent variable (y) can be estimated for known values of several independent variables (x_1, x_2, x_3, ..., x_n):

$$y = a + b_1 \cdot x_1 + b_2 \cdot x_2 + b_3 \cdot x_3 + ... + b_n \cdot x_n$$

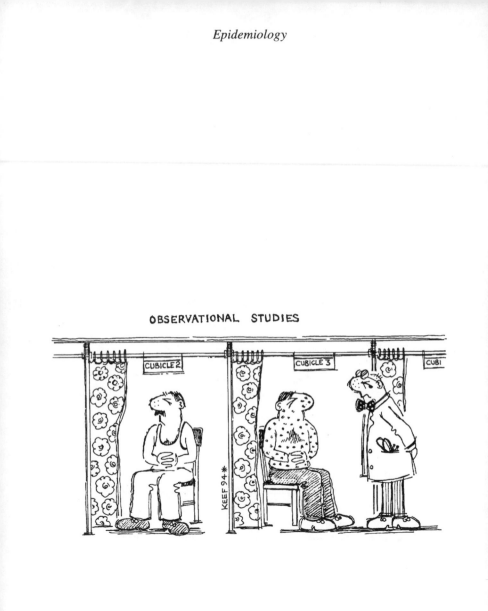

9: EPIDEMIOLOGY

Medical *epidemiology* is the study of the distribution and the determinants of diseases in human populations. It aims to:
- describe the magnitude of disease occurrence in a population (e.g. define the incidence and prevalence of illnesses)
- identify the aetiological factors responsible for particular illnesses (generally, this depends on identifying an association between a putative factor and the disease which is being studied)
- provide the information necessary to prevent, control or treat a particular disease in a specific population.

There are two broad groups of epidemiological studies used to address these aims:
- **observational** studies – described in detail in section 9.1
- **interventional** studies (clinical trials) – described in detail in section 10.1.

9.1 Observational studies

Observational studies are used to describe the distribution and aetiology of a disease. When attempting to identify possible causative factors, no intervention is made.

The number of individuals with a particular disease in a group exposed to a potential risk factor is compared to the number with the disease in a group not exposed to the factor.

Individuals cannot (usually) be randomly allocated to exposure or non-exposure; in this type of study, there is no control over who is exposed to a particular factor and who is not.

There are three major types of observational study:
- **cross-sectional (prevalence) studies** – described in detail in section 9.1.1
- **cohort studies** – described in detail in section 9.1.2
- **case-control studies** – described in detail in section 9.1.3.

9.1.1 Cross-sectional (prevalence) studies

Cross-sectional (prevalence) studies examine a defined population at a specific point in time. Such studies (surveys) are used to estimate for that

population the number of people:
* who have a particular disease, or
* who are exposed to a possible aetiological factor at that particular time.

A **case** is an individual with the characteristic of interest in the population at a given time.

The total number of cases in the population at a given time is called the **point prevalence:**

> point prevalence = number of existing cases in the population studied

The proportion of cases in the population at a given time is called the prevalence rate:

> prevalence rate = $\dfrac{\text{number of cases in the population studied}}{\text{total study population}}$

Example
A cross-sectional survey to determine the prevalence of an elevated fasting cholesterol level in men aged between 20 and 50 years in a major UK city.

Cross sectional studies provide information which is especially useful to public health workers. Such studies:
* can be used to determine the prevalence of the disease in the whole population as well as in the exposed and non-exposed groups
* are useful for examining the effects of factors which do not vary (e.g. HLA B27 status and reactive arthritis)
* are generally inexpensive and can be completed (relatively) quickly.

However:
* they have limited usefulness if the disorder is rare or of short duration since the prevalence will be small
* as the assessment of exposure and disease are made at the same time, difficulty may be experienced distinguishing between a factor which is contributing to the aetiology of a disease and one which is a consequence of having contracted the disease.

9.1.2 Cohort studies

In a **cohort/longitudinal/follow-up study**, two groups of individuals are identified:
* one group have been exposed to a potential risk factor
* the second group have not been exposed to the factor.

Both groups are followed for a pre-determined period of time. The proportions of individuals in each group found to have developed a particular characteristic (e.g. a disease of interest) are compared.

Cohorts may be defined in a variety of ways:
* birth cohorts (people born in a particular year)
* groups exposed to varying degrees to a potential toxin following an industrial accident.

The **incidence** of a condition/disease is the number of new cases occurring in the defined population in a fixed unit (period) of time:

$$\text{incidence rate} = \frac{\text{number of new cases per unit of time}}{\text{total population at risk}}$$

The incidences of a particular characteristic (disease) in a group exposed to a factor and a group not exposed to the factor are compared by computing a **relative risk:**

$$\text{relative risk} = \frac{\text{incidence rate in exposed group}}{\text{incidence rate in non-exposed group}}$$

If the value of the relative risk is:
* equal to 1, the risks for the exposed and non-exposed populations are identical
* greater than 1, the risk for the exposed group is larger than for the unexposed group
* less than 1, the risk for the exposed group is smaller than for the unexposed group.

Relative risks are best presented with their (95%) confidence interval, as this provides an indirect significance test of the Null hypothesis that the relative risk is equal to 1. If the confidence limits encompass 1 the Null hypothesis is accepted but if the limits do not include 1, the Null hypothesis is rejected and the appropriate Alternative hypothesis accepted.

Attributable risk (AR) is defined as the risk to an individual of developing the condition (disease) following exposure to a particular factor. It is computed by subtracting the incidence in the non-exposed group from the incidence in the exposed group:

AR = incidence rate in exposed group – incidence rate in non-exposed group

The **population attributable risk** (PAR) is a measure of the (negative) impact of the factor on the entire population. This is defined as:

PAR = AR x (population) prevalence of factor

Cohort studies:
- are used for the measurement of disease incidence
- can be used to determine the whole range of outcomes which can result from exposure to a specific factor (i.e. they allow the natural history of a disease to be studied)
- are useful for studying the effect of exposure to a rare event/factor.

However:
- the effect of only a limited number of exposures can be investigated
- they are not suitable for studying rare disorders/diseases
- they tend to be large, expensive and may take many years to complete
- they tend to be inflexible (a separate study is required to test a new hypothesis).

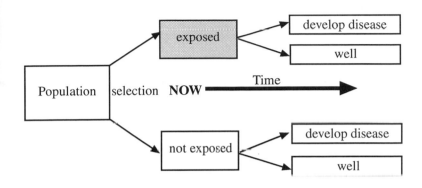

Fig. 17: The structure of a cohort study

9.1.3 Case-control studies

A **case-control** study is, in a sense, the reverse of a cohort study. In this design, two groups of individuals are again identified from a specific population:
- one group consists of patients with a particular disease **(cases)**
- the second group consists of individuals who do not have the disease **(controls)**.

Previous exposure rates to a particular (risk) factor are compared between the two groups.

The exposure rates are compared by computing an **odds ratio**:

$$\text{odds ratio} = \frac{\text{exposure rate to risk factor in cases}}{\text{exposure rate to risk factor in controls}}$$

Case-control studies are generally retrospective; cohort studies are typically prospective.

The choice of controls is usually critical. Many different types can be used, depending on the context of the study. Sources of controls include:
*   healthy individuals selected from the general population
*   patients with other (unrelated) diseases
*   family members, work colleagues, etc.

It is also crucial that the controls are similar to the cases with respect to their general characteristics (other than, of course, the disease being studied). The ideal way of achieving this is through careful **matching**, although there are often practical problems associated with this process.

Matching is carried out during the selection phase of a study. The matching procedure may consider one or several **confounding variables** (such as age, sex, HLA status, blood group, ethnic origin etc.) which may influence the prevalence of the disease being studied. Each case is paired (matched) with a control subject who is as similar to the case as possible for the confounding variable(s). The objective is that, after matching, the cases and controls will differ only with respect to one factor potentially influencing disease prevalence, namely their exposure to the risk factor(s) being studied.

Case-control studies:
*   enable a large number of factors which may contribute to the disease to be examined
*   can be used to study rare diseases
*   are generally inexpensive.

However they:
*   enable only one disease to be studied at a time
*   are not useful for studying the effects of factors/events which are rare
*   do not measure incidence.

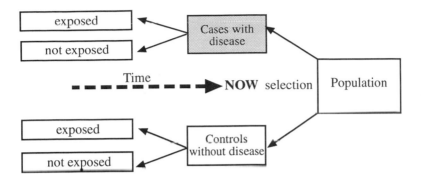

Fig. 18: The structure of a case-control study

9.2 Association and causality

Observational studies are important instruments for investigating the potential causes of a disease. They allow the **association** between a particular causative factor and the risk of developing the disease to be defined and quantified. Cohort and case-control studies allow the relative strength of a particular association to be measured (by estimating the risk of a disease developing in a group of individuals exposed to a particular risk factor relative to the risk for unexposed individuals). However:

association does not imply causation

If a study shows a statistical association between a disease and some possible causal factor, three important issues must be addressed when attempting to decide the strength of the argument in favour of the association being causal: random (Type I) error, bias and confounding.

If a large number of groups are being compared or a large number of statistical tests have to be performed, a statistically significant result is bound to occur eventually (with a conventional 5% significance level, once in every 20 tests done on average) – such false positive results occur because of **random (Type I) error**.

A poor choice of experimental design or inappropriate (e.g. non-random) patient selection methods can produce statistical **bias**. This usually occurs when there are factors influencing the measurement of either the disease or the aetiological factors which have not been properly controlled for.

Another important source of error in observational studies is **confounding**, which occurs when the exposed and non-exposed groups differ with respect to some characteristic (confounding factor) which is independent of the risk factor. If the confounding factor influences the outcome (distorting the results), the effects of the risk and confounding factors cannot be distinguished. A confounding variable is associated with the disease being studied and is different in the cases and the controls, but its effect cannot be measured directly e.g. Early studies of patients with acquired immuno-deficiency syndrome (AIDS) appeared to demonstrate an excess of amyl nitrate abuse among homosexual males with AIDS relative to those who did not have the disease. It was concluded that amyl nitrate might be causing AIDS, possibly by some toxic effect on the immune system. We now believe that AIDS is actually caused by the human immunodeficiency virus (HIV). In this instance, therefore, there was confounding between the variables HIV and amyl nitrate abuse.

All possible steps must be taken to avoid confounding. This can be done in several ways:
- it is often possible to identify potential confounding factors by referring to previously published studies/literature and standard biology
- the effect of confounding factors can sometimes be restricted (e.g. if factors such as ethnic origin or sex are possible confounders, the study could be confined to subjects who are male or who are from a single racial group)
- in intervention studies, subjects should be assigned to the control or experimental group randomly – if the total sample size is adequate, this should produce groups reasonably well balanced with respect to both known and unknown confounding factors, while coincidently reducing the risks of Type I and II errors.

Consideration of the effects of Type I errors, bias and confounding helps to determine the likelihood that any relationship observed is real. The next step is to look for any external evidence which might support the hypothesis that the relationship is causal:
- are the study findings reproducible? (i.e. does repeating the experiment, using the same or a different method of examining the same

relationship, produce a similar finding?)
- are the study findings consistent? (i.e. do similar studies on other populations produce the same findings?)
- how strong is the relationship between the variables? – a small relative risk will be statistically significant if there is a strong correlation between the variables and the sample size is sufficiently large, but the magnitude of the risk may make it clinically meaningless
- are there confounding factors which have been ignored or have not yet been identified? (i.e. is the association specific?)
- is there any evidence of a dose-response? (i.e. is the risk estimate related to the degree of exposure?)
- is the association biologically plausible?
- is the association reversible? – for example, the relationship between high blood pressure and stroke: if hypertension is treated then the risk of developing a stroke is reduced
- finally, the possibility of **reverse causation** may need to be considered.

Example
In a study of bowel cancer, patients who had carcinoma of the rectum had a high rate of new laxative prescriptions prior to the diagnosis being made – in this instance the disease is likely to be responsible for the laxative prescriptions rather than the alternative conclusion that the laxative used might be causing some bowel tumours.

If the above questions can all be answered positively, the observed association is probably a truly causative relationship between the factor and the disease. However, this only implies an increased (but possibly still small) risk – it does not imply that exposure to the factor will inevitably result in an individual developing the disease.

9.3 Rates

A **crude rate** for a particular event is the number of occurrences of the event divided by the number of individuals in the population to whom the event may occur; for example:
- the **crude attack rate** for an infection is the proportion of people exposed to infection who develop the disease in a given period of time
- the **crude annual stillbirth rate** is the number of stillbirths (born dead after 24 weeks gestation) divided by the total number of births, both live and still, in a year

- the **crude perinatal mortality rate** is the number of stillbirths and deaths in the first week of life divided by the total number of births (usually quoted per 1000 births)
- the **crude neonatal mortality rate** is the number of deaths in the first four weeks of life divided by the number of live births (again usually reported per 1000 live births)
- the **crude infant mortality rate** is the number of deaths in the first year of life divided by the number of live births (again per 1000 live births)
- the **crude maternal mortality rate** is the number of deaths of mothers attributed to pregnancy and delivery by the number of births (usually expressed in deaths per 100,000 births).

The **crude mortality rate (CMR)** for the entire population of a country for a particular year is given by the total number of deaths occurring in that year divided by the population of the country at the mid-point of the year. This figure is usually multiplied by 1000 to give the CMR for a particular year per 1000 individuals.

Rates do not have to be restricted to entire populations. For example, mortality rates may vary by age. Thus:
- the **age-specific mortality rate (ASMR)** is defined as the number of deaths occurring in the age group of interest divided by the total number of individuals in the population falling into that age group – as for CMR, this ratio is usually expressed per 1000 individuals.

When making comparisons between death rates in different parts of the country, the use of crude rates could be misleading. Differences in demographic factors, such as age distribution, across the country must be taken into account. **Standardised rates** are used for this purpose:
- the **standardised mortality ratio (SMR)** for a particular time period is defined as the ratio of the observed death rate in the study (index) population to the expected death rate:

SMR = (observed deaths in study population/total expected deaths) x 100

- the number of expected deaths is calculated from the age-specific mortality rates in the standard population
- the population used as the standard population is arbitrary and will depend on the purpose of the study
- SMRs may be calculated for particular communities, occupations, etc.

and may be used as outcome measures in clinical trials
- if the SMR is greater than 100 then that population has an increased mortality rate compared to the standard
- if the SMR is smaller than 100 then that population has a decreased mortality rate compared to the standard.

10: INTERVENTIONAL STUDIES/CLINICAL TRIALS

10.1 Interventional studies/clinical trials

In an **interventional** study, the investigators have control over who is exposed and who is not exposed to a particular factor/intervention (e.g. a treatment such as a vaccine).

Such studies generally take the form of a **randomised controlled clinical trial (RCT)**. RCTs are widely considered to be the 'gold standard' method for obtaining evidence about the effect of a treatment/intervention.

An interventional study must be properly designed if valid conclusions are to be drawn. No amount of statistical manipulation of the results can salvage a badly designed study. Arguably, a poorly designed and conducted clinical trial is unethical as:
* resources are wasted
* patients may be exposed to the risks of treatment without the justification of advancing medical knowledge
* clinicians may be misled on the relative merits of a new treatment.

A good trial design will optimise the chances of accurately estimating the relative efficacy of the treatments being compared by avoiding potential sources of bias and by controlling for confounding variables.

Randomised controlled clinical trials always consist of:
* one or more **treatment groups**, consisting of patients or volunteers who receive the new test treatment(s)
* one or more **control groups**, consisting of patients receiving no treatment, a placebo treatment or a standard treatment (of established efficacy).

One well designed study of adequate size should be sufficient to establish the clinical worth of a new treatment. If further studies are to be carried out, there must be:
* sufficient doubt about the effectiveness of the new treatment to justify not giving it to the **control** group
* sufficient confidence in the potential effectiveness and safety of the new therapy to justify giving it to the individuals in the **treatment** group.

10.2 Study protocols

The most important document in a clinical trial is the **study protocol**. This fully details the purpose, design and methodology of the study. Arguably, a new investigator should be able to fully participate in the administration of a study having read the protocol. The major components of a good study protocol are outlined in the rest of this section.

10.2.1 Objectives

The purpose of the study (the question which the trial is designed to answer) must be clearly stated. Ideally, this should be supported by a brief rationale and literature survey. Where appropriate, the objectives should be stated as Null and Alternative hypotheses (section 7.1).

10.2.2 Design

Uncontrolled clinical trials. All subjects receive the same test treatment. This design is mainly used in preliminary studies to assess tolerable doses, toxicity, etc. It is not suitable for assessing efficacy, but may be useful in establishing the absence of clinical efficacy or the presence of undesirable adverse reactions.

Controlled (randomised) trials (RCTs). These are used mainly to compare a treatment group with a control group (section 10.1). Control groups take several forms:
- no treatment if spontaneous improvement is likely
- a placebo if there is no widely accepted standard treatment
- the standard treatment – this should be the best currently available, otherwise the trial does little to help decide whether the new treatment is a useful clinical advance.

Two main types of design are used for RCTs.

Group comparative studies. Each subject is allocated to just one of the test interventions; the control and treatment groups contain different individuals. Comparisons are made between the groups ('between-subjects'). Interpretation of the study results depends on the groups being comparable with respect to important (possibly confounding) characteristics.

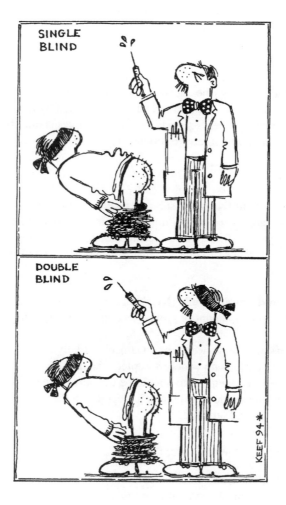

Cross-over studies. Each subject receives several (often all) of the interventions being compared in a randomised sequence. Subjects act as their own controls and comparisons are made 'within-subjects'. This design is optimal for treatments which have short term benefits in patients with a chronic but relatively stable disease. The validity of the comparisons is dependent on an adequate washout period being allowed between treatments; otherwise effects carry-over between treatment periods and introduce confounding of effects can occur. An assessment of the 'stability of the disease' both before and after the treatments is also useful, achieved by using 'run-in' and 'run-out' periods respectively.

Sequential trial design. The results obtained from each subject who completes the study are continuously assessed to determine if the current (observed) difference between the treatments has achieved statistical significance. They have the advantage that no assumption about the size of the difference in the effectiveness of two treatments is needed (see section 7.3). For a given effect, smaller numbers of patients will be needed for a sequential relative to a standard design, but the chance of a Type I error is increased. This design requires the use of complex statistical methods outside the scope of this book.

10.2.3 Blinding of assessments

If either the patient or the investigator knows which intervention the patient is receiving, this knowledge may bias the investigator's assessment of response. This is a particular problem if the measure of response has a subjective element (e.g. global assessment of well-being).

The risk of bias is greatly reduced if treatments are allocated **blind**:
- if only the patient has no knowledge of the intervention, the study is **single blind**
- if neither the patient nor the investigator knows the identity of the intervention, the study is **double blind**
- if the patient, the investigator and the person analysing the study results are all unaware of the intervention being used, the study is **triple blind**.

Blinded studies are not always practical. An alternative is to have a method of assessing outcome which is independent of the investigator. In this situation, the person carrying out the assessment of the effects of the interventions is different from the clinician responsible for each patient's care.

A code-break must be available at all times in the case of emergency (e.g. a patient overdoses on their study medication).

10.2.4 Definition of study population

Patients to be studied. These are usually enshrined in a set of inclusion and exclusion criteria for eligibility for inclusion in the trial. Careful consideration is needed to ensure that the most appropriate population is studied. The applicability of the study findings depends on the population studied. The findings hold only for the population on which the study was conducted. The more selected and particular the trial population is, the less the results will be generally applicable. **Extrapolation to other populations may not be valid**.

Examples
A hospital based study may not produce findings pertinent to patients attending their General Practitioner, and vice-versa.
If elderly patients or women who are (likely to become) pregnant are excluded, how will this affect the applicability of the results?

Disease definition. Often difficult, particularly in multi-centre studies; the definition should be comprehensive, including diagnostic criteria, permissible severity of disease, potential risk factors, length of history allowed, influence of previous/concomitant therapy taken, etc.

Definition of treatment. This should include details of the dose, formulation and route of administration. The protocol for altering the dose if side-effects develop must be detailed. A list of other medication permitted during the study period is required, as is a description of the method used to assess the level of compliance for each patient.

Methods of evaluation/measurement. The evaluation of the effects of the test interventions should involve methods which are standard, as objective as possible, and reproducible; ideally, they should all have been validated. A primary outcome measure should be defined which determines what constitutes a treatment success and failure. The circumstances when a patient should be withdrawn should be defined as should how such an event would be handled in the analysis of the study results. Some trials allow replacement of drop-outs if they fulfil previously defined criteria.

10.2.5 Allocation to treatment

THE DESIGN OF A CONTROLLED TRIAL MUST GIVE CAREFUL
CONSIDERATION TO ELIMINATING SELECTION BIAS. THIS CAN
BE ACHIEVED BY ALLOCATING SUBJECTS TO THE
INTERVENTION GROUPS USING A RANDOM PROCESS

Simple randomisation ensures that each patient has an equal chance of
being assigned to each intervention group. Allocation is determined by
random numbers (usually generated by a computer); this is equivalent to
tossing a coin or throwing a die. Other methods of allocating to treatment,
such as using the subject's date of birth or hospital number, may appear
random, but rarely are – these should never be used.

Stratified randomisation ensures that patients with common potential
confounding factors are equally distributed between the study groups. The
patients are divided into sub-groups (strata) defined by these factors and
simple random allocation is carried out within each separately. The
proportion of subjects selected from each stratum is determined so as to
ensure that each is of sufficient size to be analysed; in some studies, small
rarely occurring strata may need be over represented.

Examples
1. To ensure that the patients allocated to two study groups were similar
with respect to age, separate randomisation processes were used for the
following three age strata:

    18 – 39 years   40 – 54 years   55 – 70 years

2. To ensure that the patients allocated to two study groups were similar
with respect to age and sex distribution, separate randomisation processes
were used for the following strata:

males 18 – 39 years	males 40 – 54 years	males 55 – 70 years
females 18 – 39 years	females 40 – 54 years	females 55 – 70 years

Blocked randomisation is used to ensure that allocation to each study
group is balanced at regular points throughout a study. Blocking is done
within all strata present.

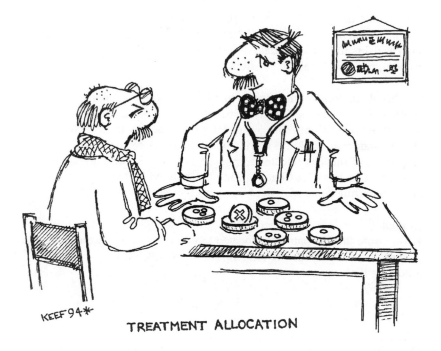

TREATMENT ALLOCATION

Example

A simple randomisation process, used for a study to compare a control and a new treatment, was blocked in groups of four. In practice, allocation was manipulated within consecutive blocks of four subjects so that, within each block, two patients were allocated to receive the new treatment and two to receive the control.

If all participants in the study are available at its start, **matching** can be used to achieve comparable groups. Subjects are paired who are similar to each other with respect to the main potential confounding variables (e.g. sex, age, disease severity). One member of each pair is randomly allocated to the new treatment and the other to the control group.

Balanced allocation of patients with common potential confounding characteristics can also be achieved using a computer-based method of allocation called **minimisation**. This uses a simple mathematical algorithm to determine, on the basis of the characteristics of all patients currently entered into the study, the intervention group to which a newly presenting subject should be allocated.

10.2.6 Power/sample size

It is possible that if the sample size for a study is:

* **too small**, a clinically significant difference between the treatments may not be established as statistically significant and all patients admitted to the new treatment may have been exposed to increased risk for no satisfactory scientific outcome
* **too large**, the 'surplus' patients admitted to the new treatment may have been exposed to unnecessary risk.

Both situations are, arguably, unethical.

The optimum sample size for a study should be determined, based on the desired power level. Simple formulae exist for most commonly used study designs, based on the following information (see also section 7.3):

* the smallest difference in the primary outcome measure considered clinically significant
* the (estimated) variability of the primary outcome measure
* the acceptable levels for the Type I and Type II error rates.

The smaller the (clinically significant) difference that the study is required to establish as statistically significant, the larger the optimum sample size is likely to be.

Lack of attention to power levels can lead to misleading conclusions. For example, the early studies of streptokinase on survival following myocardial infarction failed to detect any statistically significant effects. These trials, however, involved only a few hundred patients. When larger and, by definition, more powerful trials were conducted, a statistically significant increase in survival was detected. The size of the increase in survival was **small in percentage terms**, but **clinically extremely important**.

10.2.7 Statistical methods

These should be stated in general terms.

The whole of the original study sample should be included in the report of the final statistical evaluation. Patients who withdraw should be accounted for (incidence of side effects, failure to respond, etc.). Bias may be introduced if subjects who fail to complete the trial (for whatever reason) are excluded from the analysis. Consequently, an analysis of outcome by **intention to treat** should be carried out in addition to any evaluations based just on those patients who complete the trial.

The statistical analysis should be restricted to the stated study objectives. The more significance tests that are carried out, the greater the chance of a Type I error occurring. Apparently significant results unearthed by 'data-dredging' should be regarded with the utmost scepticism, and should be subjected to a confirmatory, prospective study.

10.2.8 Dissemination of findings

Many grant-awarding bodies now require a detailed account of how the results of a research project will be disseminated before they will offer funding. In general terms, it is no longer sufficient to merely publish the findings in a suitable reputable medical journal. A more extensive strategy is now required, including presentation at appropriate local, national and (where appropriate) international conferences/meetings.

Positive studies showing differences which are both statistically and clinically significant have a much greater chance of being published than (potentially equally important) negative studies; this is often referred to as **publication bias**.

10.3 Meta-analysis

Meta-analysis is a somewhat controversial statistical method used to combine the results from several similar studies. The technique attempts to:

- increase the statistical power of any common conclusions from the studies (and hence improve the confidence of any estimates which have been obtained)
- resolve uncertainty if the original trials disagree
- analyse aspects of the trials which were not possible when each trial was examined individually.

A meta-analysis is often used when the results of the available published trials appear to be contradictory; however, it may be used when:

- the results of the definitive randomised controlled trial are not yet available, or
- it is not possible, practical or ethical to conduct a definitive trial.

For a meta-analysis to be valid:

- the populations from which the study samples were drawn should be similar
- the design methods employed in each should be similar
- all suitable studies (*including any not published*) should be included in the calculations.

It is rare for these conditions to be met completely.

This is a brief resumé of the main points to be considered when reading the report of a clinical trial or experiment. No study can be perfect, so each question should be considered from the point of view of reasonable practice rather than in absolute terms.

There are five main questions which should be addressed when assessing a report.

What question (objective) was the study attempting to answer?

What experiment was carried out?
The most important consideration is the adequacy of the experimental design. This can be broken down into the following sub-questions:
- was the type of study carried out appropriate for the study objectives?
- was the study population adequately defined and relevant?
- how were the subjects selected - is there a possibility of selection bias?
- what control interventions were used - were they appropriate and comparable with the treatment group - were they a proper random sample - were the study procedures exactly the same for all groups (except for the actual intervention given)?
- were the methods and measurements clearly defined - were there any potential confounding variables which were not considered - could the assessment methods have introduced bias and, if so, was this adequately dealt with?
- do the methods used seem reproducible?

What results were obtained?
Specifically:
- do the results make sense and are they consistent?
- are the results given in sufficient detail for a reader of the report to reach their own (if necessary different) conclusions?
- have appropriate statistical methods been applied, properly reported and interpreted?
- have all subjects who were admitted to the study and randomised been accounted for - if the drop-out (attrition) rate was high, does this affect the conclusions that can be drawn - have the results been analysed on an intention-to-treat basis?

Have the study objectives been met?

Most importantly:

- is the result for the primary study objective statistically significant – have the summary statistics been presented appropriately (preferably with confidence limits)?
- could the result obtained be explained by other factors than a real difference between the interventions (selection bias, effects of confounding variables, etc.)?
- does the result make sense when compared with findings from previously published studies – are the conclusions and findings related directly to the original study objective or are they a consequence of 'data dredging'?

Is the result relevant to ordinary clinical practice?

Specifically:

- can the results of the study be applied to the sort of population the reader has clinical responsibility for? (e.g. the results of a drug trial involving mainly young subjects with no concomitant diseases cannot necessarily be applied to an elderly population with numerous other ailments)
- if the results are presented in the form of relative risks, are they also presented in more directly relevant terms (e.g. *absolute* reduction in risk, *actual* improvement in blood pressure, number needed to treat, etc.)?

12: SAMPLE MULTIPLE CHOICE QUESTIONS

Mark your answers in the box provided.

1. **The following are true:**

    ❏   A   the annual prevalence of a condition reflects the number of new
             cases reported annually
    ❏   B   studies with a cross-sectional design are useful when attempting to
             detect associations between risk factors and disease
    ❏   C   in a frequency distribution, the mode is the most frequently
             observed value
    ❏   D   if a measurement has a skewed distribution, then the mean and
             mode are always different
    ❏   E   the standard deviation of a population may be smaller than the
             standard error of a sample mean from that population

2. **A study examines the stature of school children. The conclusion**
    states that there is a relation between the heights of siblings shown
    by the tendency of tall boys to have tall sisters ($r = +0.57$, $p <$
    0.001). The following are correct:

    ❏   A   the symbol r represents the correlation coefficient
    ❏   B   as $r > 0$, a negative correlation has been demonstrated
    ❏   C   the value p indicates the result is highly significant
    ❏   D   the result means that the sisters of tall boys are likely to be taller
             than the sisters of short boys
    ❏   E   the statement $p < 0.001$ suggests too few measurements were made

3. **In the clinical trial of a new drug**

    ❏   A   randomisation ensures that a patient has an equal chance of being
             assigned to each of the treatment groups
    ❏   B   a small number of patients implies that the trial is likely to be
             statistically powerful
    ❏   C   the placebo response can generally be ignored
    ❏   D   a stratified random allocation is important when small numbers of
             patients are to be used in the trial
    ❏   E   the number of patients who withdraw because of side-effects
             should be included in the analysis

4. **If a set of observations are Normally distributed the following are true:**

❏ A the median value will be less than the mean
❏ B 2.5% of the observations will have numerical values which are smaller than the mean value minus 1.96 standard deviations
❏ C the standard deviation is a measure of how accurately the calculated mean approaches the true population mean
❏ D Student unpaired t-test may be used to compare this set of observations with those from a different group of individuals provided they are also normally distributed
❏ E the modal value is equal to the mean

5. **The average heights of two groups of subjects are compared and are stated to be significantly different (p < 0.05). The following are true:**

❏ A Student paired t-test should have been used to calculate p
❏ B the likelihood that this result may have arisen by chance alone is less than one time in twenty
❏ C if the t-test is used the number of degrees of freedom is the total number of observations in both groups minus two
❏ D even if the difference is large it has not reached conventional levels of statistical significance
❏ E for the result to be valid the groups need to have been chosen randomly

6. **The median is used in preference to the arithmetic mean when**

❏ A the variance is large
❏ B the sample size is small
❏ C the observations are from a population with a skewed distribution
❏ D observer error is likely to be large
❏ E the standard deviation is to be calculated

7. In a single blind clinical trial of a new treatment

❑ A the null hypothesis is true if there is a statistically significant difference between the responses of the treatment and placebo groups

❑ B the patients should be allocated randomly to the treatment and control groups

❑ C stratified random allocation of patients is essential if the groups are large

❑ D a Type I error has occurred if the Null hypothesis is wrongly rejected

❑ E neither the patient nor the assessor know which treatment an individual is receiving

8. For Pearson's coefficient of correlation (r) the following are correct:

❑ A the value of r lies between -1 and +1

❑ B if r = 0.1, this excludes a statistically significant correlation between the variables

❑ C if r is negative, as one variable increases the other decreases

❑ D one of the variables needs to be Normally distributed

❑ E r can be used to predict one variable from a value of the other

9. In the trial of a new antibiotic the cure rates appeared to improve when compared to the old treatment regimen ($\chi^2 = 7.2$ with one degree of freedom; $p < 0.01$). The following are true:

❑ A the improvement with the new treatment must be clinically significant

❑ B to calculate χ^2 the cure rates must be converted to percentages

❑ C the conclusion that there is a significant difference may be invalid if there was a significant difference in the ages of the two treatment groups

❑ D the trial implies that a difference in response of 7.2 times was observed

❑ E the results may have occurred by chance one time in twenty

10. The following are true for within-patient comparisons:

❏ A usually fewer patients are needed than for between-patient comparisons

❏ B they may have an advantage when examining the effects of long acting drugs

❏ C they may be used to analyse possible short-term relief of symptoms in chronic conditions

❏ D they are free from carry-over effects

❏ E they cannot be randomised

SAMPLE MULTIPLE CHOICE QUESTION ANSWERS

1.   **Answers: C D**

The annual prevalence of a condition defines the annual incidence of the condition. Associations between risk factors and disease must be examined using an appropriate longitudinal design. The standard error is equal to the standard deviation divided by the square root of the sample size. By definiton, therefore, the standard deviation cannot be smaller than the standard error.

2.   **Answers: A C D**

A positive value of r indicates a **positive** association between the heights of siblings. The fact that the value of p is so very small indicates that the sample size was adequate to detect a statistically significant relationship between the heights of siblings.

3.   **Answers: A D E**

In general terms, the larger the sample size, the greater the statistical power of the study. Reducing the number of patients will tend to reduce the power. The real clinical effect of the new drug can only be estimated if an appropriate adjustment is made for any placebo effect. The response in the patients allocated to the new drug will be equal to the real effect of the drug plus (a proportion of) the placebo effect.

4.   **Answers: B D E**

If a set of observations are Normally distributed, the mean and median should be equal. The standard deviation is a measure of the extent to which the sample observations vary (distribute) around the sample mean.

5.   **Answers: B C E**

The groups in this study consist of different subjects and so they are statistically independent. Assuming the heights are Normally distributed, the Student unpaired t-test should be used. $p < 0.05$ indicates that the difference is statistically significant at the conventional 5% level.

6.   **Answer: C**

The arithmetic mean should be used for continuous observations which can be assumed to follow or approximate a Normal distribution. If the observations follow a skewed distribution, the median is more appropriate. Considerations of sample size and variation/standard deviation/standard error are irrelevant.

7.   **Answers: B D**
If the difference between the treatment and placebo groups is statistically significant, the Null hypothesis is rejected and the Alternative hypothesis is accepted as being true. Although stratifying samples for important confounding variables is always sound science, it becomes **less** important as the sample size increases. In a single blind trial, only the patient does not know which treatment has been allocated.

8.   **Answers: A C D**
A value of r as small as 0.1 is unlikely to be statistically significant, but if the sample size is increased sufficiently, significance will eventually be reached. r only measures the strength of the association between variables, It tells nothing about the mathematical form of the relationship.

9.   **Answer: C**
Although the improvement in the cure rate is **statistically** significant, the cure rates may in fact be sufficiently similar that the difference between them is not **clinically** significant. Calculation of the χ^2 must only be done using the raw frequencies, **never** from the group percentages. The value of the test statistic gives no direct information about the size of the difference in cure rates. If the Null hypothesis is true, the observed difference in cure rates would occur by chance less than one time in a hundred.

10.   **Answers: A C**
Patient comparison studies where patients are using long acting drugs require long treatment periods and consequently compliance can become a problem if each patient has to undergo two or more such periods. Within-subject/cross-over studies are often prone to carry-over effects and may require long wash-out periods between treatments. The order in which each patient receives the treatments being compared **must** be randomised.

INDEX

PASTEST COURSES

PASTEST: the key to exam success, the key to your future.
PasTest is dedicated to helping doctors to pass their professional examinations. We have 25 years of specialist experience in medical education and over 3000 doctors attend our revision courses each year.

Experienced lecturers:
Many of our lecturers are also examiners and teach in a lively and interesting way in order to:
✓   reflect current trends in exams
✓   give plenty of mock exam practice
✓   provide essential advice on exam technique

Outstanding accelerated learning:
Our up-to-date and relevant course material includes MCQs, colour slides, X-rays, ECGs, EEGs, clinical cases, data interpretations, mock exams, vivas and extensive course notes which provide:
✓   hundreds of high quality questions with detailed answers and explanations
✓   succinct notes, diagrams and charts

Personal attention:
Active participation is encouraged on these courses, so in order to give personal tuition and to answer individual questions our course numbers are limited. Book early to avoid disappointment.

Choice of courses:
PasTest has developed a wide range of high quality interactive courses in different cities around the UK to suit your individual needs.

What other students have said about our courses:
'Absolutely brilliant - I would not have passed without it! Thank you.'
Dr Charitha Rajapakse, London.
'Excellent, enjoyable, extremely hard work but worth every penny.'
Dr Helen Binns, Oxford.

For further details contact:
PasTest, Egerton Court, Parkgate Estate, Knutsford, Cheshire WA16 8DX, UK.

Telephone: 01565 755226   **Fax: 01565 650264**
e-mail: pastest@dial.pipex.com
web site: http:\\www.pastest.co.uk